HEALING WITH EASE

RICK HALL D.C.

For Ellie, Courtney and Julianne,
And for
June and Bob

With Love and Gratitude

ACKNOWLEDGMENTS

There have been so many chiropractors who have helped and guided me throughout my life. Some are teachers from New York Chiropractic College, and others from post-graduate training. Many are friends and family, and I am so grateful to all these wonderful doctors for their love, insight, their case histories and permission to share some of their stories.

Alice Behr, DC

Kate Brown, DC

Nancy Cagen, DC

Steve Cagen, DC

Anthony Caliendo, DC

Frank DiGiacomo, DC

James Dubel, DC

Donald Epstein, DC

Joseph Flesia, DC

Alan Furman, DC

Chuck Gibson. DC

Reggie Gold. DC

Bob Hall, DC

Barbara Harvey, DC

Tedd Koren, DC

Frank Langilotti, DC

Glen Mark, DC

Nancy Mark, DC

B.J. Palmer, DC

D.D. Palmer, DC

James Parker, DC

Bradley Rauch, DC

Chuck Ribley, DC

Guy Riekeman, DC

Jason Schwartz, DC

Jim Sigafoose, DC

Michael Stern, DC

Joseph Strauss, DC

Clay Thompson, DC

Steven Weiss, DC

Thank you to the following proofreaders and editors for their patience, attention to detail and thoughtful suggestions:

Jay Batterman	Glenn Jochum*
Janet Brock-Kraebel	Nancy Kardwell
Vito DeLaurentis	Nancy Kongoletis
Liz DeTour	Steve Masciangelo
Krystal Foster	Paul Matthews
Ellie Hall	Anthony Mitarotondo, MD
June Hall	Frank Notaro
Michael John Hall	Susan Worth

*An extra thank you to Glenn Jochum for his many hours of editorial work.

Thank you to Brianna Michelle Bruno for her beautiful cover artwork and permission to reproduce it.

Thank you to The New Renaissance and Drs. Joseph Flesia, Guy Riekeman, Kevin Pallis and Ed Plentz for permission to reprint the Five Components of the Vertebral Subluxation Complex.

And finally, a huge heartfelt thank you to my family for their patience and understanding regarding my deep need to write this story about chiropractic.

INTRODUCTION

Above the desk where I write is a quote by Kurt Vonnegut, Jr.

Find a subject you care about and which in your heart you feel others should care about. It is the genuine caring, and not your games with language, which will be the most compelling and seductive element in your style.

The purpose of this book is to enlighten and inform people about the most misunderstood health care profession in the world today – chiropractic. This book will help you understand what chiropractic *is*, what it is *not*, and how it can help you and your family live healthier and happier lives.

Due to more than 100 years of propaganda, slander and misinformation, many people today hear the word *chiropractic* and think they know what it is, but my experience has shown me that they really don't. They've heard and read a little bit about it, and maybe even experienced it. But rare is the person who truly knows what chiropractic is about. Because of these preconceptions and misconceptions, I have found it very challenging to explain chiropractic in a five-minute talk or even in an hour lay lecture. So I decided to write a story about the words and ideas that inspired me and others to become chiropractors. The case histories used as examples are based on true experiences. They come from my own practice as well as from other chiropractors. Names have been changed to protect privacy. I am grateful for their stories and permission to use them.

This book is about one of the most unknown, misunderstood and neglected concepts in health care – the function of the spine and nervous system and their relationship to health and vitality. And if it motivates even one parent to bring his or her child to a chiropractor, I have done my job.

I understand that not everyone cares about health and longevity. Some people just want relief from their pain or condition. If your objective is pain relief, this book will still help you. If you want to understand your pain, symptoms, condition or disease better, or perhaps why you haven't been able to heal or recover from an injury or illness, this book will definitely help you even more. If your goal is to regain your health or to be as healthy and alive as possible, then you will gain much from reading and understanding the words within these pages.

When I originally wrote the book, I added a long bibliography with suggested readings and references to dozens of published scientific papers. I decided to forego the list and let my words speak for themselves. It's easy to find information these days. Instead, I appeal to your reason and common sense. Similarly, I turned the book from an authoritative, instructional and sterile textbook into a story with dialogue designed to get you to think.

I believe that truth cannot be taught, but must be caught, and it is my sincere hope that you catch the simple, beautiful and profound truths within chiropractic.

As you read, I ask you to challenge your thinking and logic. Let go of your preconceptions and judgments as much as possible, think simply and sensibly, and have an open heart and mind. Thank you.

Rick Hall, D.C.
September, 2015

A mind that is stretched to a new idea never returns to its original dimensions.

Oliver Wendell Holmes

1

The old wooden rowboat creaked and groaned. It was Mike's turn to row. I sat peacefully in the bow, my gaze shifting slowly back and forth between the multi-colored sunrise and our catch of the morning, eight huge blue-claw crabs and three eels. I was a 10-year-old boy in a creek with my 12-year-old brother and no one else around.

At my feet were two buckets teeming with action. The eels fascinated me, but were much too slimy to play with. The blue-claws, very much alive in the other bucket, offered some challenging games. Some of them had claws bigger than my hands, so like any foolish young boy, I'd either pick one up and see how close to my nose I could hold it, or just flick my fingers at them in the bucket, challenging them to grab me. This was a great game until one latched on to a finger. Once you experienced the power of a blue-claw crab, you knew never to let one get too close to anything it could grab.

About five minutes away from our dock, while playing with the crabs, my chest tightened and my breathing shortened. Agitated, I asked Mike to row faster. He started to ask why, but with one look at my face he knew. Within 30 seconds, I could hardly breathe. I had left my inhaler on my night table. Mike rowed as fast as he could.

When we reached the dock, we saw a stocky man with thick, fuzzy sideburns – my Uncle Earl. He bellowed out, "How are my two favorite nephews on this beautiful day?" Although I hadn't seen him in nearly two years, he was easy to recognize. He looked like a shorter and wider version of my dad. He and dad had the same piercing blue eyes and warm smiles, but he and dad didn't get along too well, which is why I rarely saw him. He lived out west, but during the summer they shared this big bay front house they inherited from my grandparents. On this day, I couldn't smile or return his greeting. His big grin quickly changed to concern when he saw me. He grabbed and tied the bowline, and helped me off the boat. I was choking and my face was beet-red. I was nearly in a state of panic. He carried me to the house.

Inside, mom got me my inhaler, gave me two pills and gently rubbed my forehead. I'd had these severe asthma attacks for about five years now. Dad was a pediatrician, so he'd taken me to half a dozen specialists, and I'd tried just about every kind of medicine available. Nothing helped though, other than the temporary relief offered by the steroid inhaler. Recently, the attacks were more frequent and more severe.

Uncle Earl knocked quietly and walked into my bedroom while mom tried desperately to soothe my fear. After questioning mom about my asthma, he asked if he could check my spine. He explained to us that sometimes, due to stress or trauma, the bones of the spine move out of place a bit, irritating the spinal cord and nerves. He told us that asthma was a neurological condition because the nervous system is what controls dilation and constriction of the bronchi and bronchioles. He told me that what he did all day long at his job was check people's spines and make adjustments to relieve the pressure on the nervous system. He said there is a miraculous wisdom that runs the body, and that it uses the nervous system to control and coordinate everything that occurs in the body. Mom was unsure, but knew the fear and treatments I'd been enduring, and decided to allow Uncle Earl to check my spine.

He found a very painful spot on the left side of my neck. "This top bone in your neck is really stuck, Adam. If it's OK with you, I'd like to adjust it from left to right," he said. Mom looked at him as though he had a loaded gun pointed at my head, but I said "OK". He grabbed my head and neck in his thick, hairy hands, smiled and asked me to look up at him. At that moment, he tugged on my neck and I heard a loud crack. Mom let out a short "Oh, my goodness" and stared intently at me, as though she expected me to die on the spot. As surprised as I was at the loud noise, I was even more surprised that it didn't hurt at all.

I fell asleep and woke up three hours later. I felt great, and I never had another asthma attack.

I never got to thank Uncle Earl. When I woke up after he had adjusted my neck, he was gone. I found out a few years later that he and my dad had a huge argument that day. They haven't spoken since, so I haven't seen my uncle for more than a decade.

The timid never find true love and happiness,
but the bold do.

Paul Twitchell

2

It was the middle of June, and I packed my Chevy pick-up with a few weeks' worth of clothes, camping and hiking gear, and my guitar. I had just graduated from college, and was accepted and excited to start medical school in the fall. I had a few weeks to travel, and I planned to see some of this magnificent country.

The trip was filled with wonderful people, phenomenal scenery, and lots of great music. I camped out in beautiful national and state parks, and saw moose, bear, elk, deer, buffalo, coyotes, owls, hawks and eagles. I played guitar and sang around campfires with other travelers from all over the world.

Every night, weather permitting, I loved to lie on my back and gaze at the brilliant stars in the night sky. Often my thoughts were of dad and Uncle Earl. I realized that in many families there are often harsh words that lead to broken relationships, but the few times I asked my dad about his brother, he rarely told me much. He would say things like, "I don't want his name mentioned in this house," or "He's crazy. There's nothing to talk about."

Mom told me stories about how close dad and Uncle Earl were as kids. For many years, they played baseball and football together. They loved making music together, dad on piano and Uncle Earl on guitar. Even after dad graduated medical school and became a pediatrician, they were as close as brothers could be.

Things changed when Uncle Earl decided to go to chiropractic college. He and dad would argue day after day about the validity, and to dad, the absurdity of chiropractic. Dad would call Earl a witch doctor, and Uncle Earl would call dad a closed-minded fool. Gradually, their closeness turned to bitterness and disdain, and on my tenth birthday, the day Uncle Earl adjusted me, they stopped talking altogether. Uncle Earl never returned to Long Island. Mom and my Aunt Cathy still remain friends, and talk on the phone once or twice a month, mostly keeping each other up to date on the lives of their children and grandchildren.

One night in Yellowstone National Park, I heard a band of coyotes howling and made a spur-of-the-moment decision to visit Uncle Earl, in spite of dad's warnings not to. I wanted to see for myself just how crazy my uncle was, so early the next morning I packed up my gear and headed south from Yellowstone to Southold Springs, Colorado, where my uncle now lived.

On the second of July, a little after noon, I drove into the charming little town of Southold Springs. Flowers bloomed, and huge shade trees lined the streets. In the heart of town, I noticed a sign outside a classic gray clapboard Victorian that read *Earl Hale, D.C., Catherine Hale, D.C., Emily Hale, D.C., Megan Thompson, D.C., and James Thompson, D.C., Chiropractors.* These were my aunt and uncle, my two cousins, and Megan's husband, Jim.

I was nervous, and not quite ready to see anyone yet, so I drove past the big house and parked a few blocks up in front of *The Coronet*, a rural luncheonette. Inside to my left were eight stools along a counter, and to the right were six booths. In between were roughly a dozen tables. A teenaged, gum-chewing waitress named Jennie led me to a booth with torn blue vinyl seats and a newspaper-sized menu.

I ordered a tuna sandwich and a chocolate shake, and asked Jennie if she knew of any cheap hotels in town. Just in case my Uncle Earl was *really* crazy, I wanted to sleep in a safe place. She told me of a reasonably priced bed and breakfast about a mile outside of town. After lunch, I handed Jennie my credit card, and upon seeing my name, she quickly asked, "Are you related to Dr. Earl Hale?" I told her I was his nephew, and asked her how she knew him. "I've been going to him my whole life," she replied.

"*Going* to him?" I asked. She looked at me quizzically and said, "You know, getting adjusted." She didn't look weird to me, so I asked her why she got adjusted. "To be healthy. Everybody does." *Everybody does? What in the world does that mean?* I thought. "Do you have a back problem?" I asked. "No silly, I just go every week." I couldn't understand this, so I pressed, "But *why*?" She looked a little frustrated with me, but answered, "I don't know. I just always have. Since I was a baby."

I left the luncheonette, got in my pick-up, and pulled into a nearby gas station. When the elderly gas attendant looked at my credit card, the same thing happened.

"You related to Doc Earl?"

"Yes, he's my uncle."

"He and I have been good friends for almost 20 years. We fish together up in Eagle River every summer. You must be Ward's son."

"How did you know that?" I asked.

"Oh, he told me of his brother and their falling out. I'm sorry. Families should stick together."

I wanted to learn more about my dad and his relationship with his brother, so I asked him what he knew about their "falling out".

"Well, mostly that your dad didn't understand chiropractic, but you better ask your uncle about all that."

"Don't tell me you get adjusted too, do you?"

"Every week. And my wife, kids and grandkids, too."

I thanked him and drove off, still a bit baffled. I stopped in a convenience store to get a few things. I asked the clerk, "Do you know Dr. Earl Hale?" "Yes", he said, "I see his daughter Emily every week."

This seemed so odd to me. "Why do you go every week? Do you have a back problem?"

He answered, "Well, I used to, but not anymore. When something works, you stick with it."

I smiled, paid my bill, and walked out in disbelief. *What a strange place,* I thought. I drove about a mile up a long, winding mountain road to the B & B.

*How we do one thing in life
is how we do everything.*

T. Harv Eker

3

In fewer than five minutes, I pulled into a long driveway that led to the Southold Springs Hilltop Bed and Breakfast. It was a large white house with a wrap-around porch and two big Newfoundland dogs lying lazily on the front lawn. There was an orchard in the back yard, and about a dozen gigantic evergreen trees around the front and sides of the house. For all I knew, they could have been redwoods. They each looked more than 100 feet tall.

The hand-carved, wooden sign over the front door read, *Sam and Edna Sprague, Proprietors*. Edna Sprague greeted me at the front door. She looked very old and seemed quite proper. Her white hair was neatly tied in a bun and her blue plaid dress was crisply pressed. She asked me quite a few questions as we walked inside. *Where was I from? What was I doing in Southold Springs? What kind of work did I do?*

When she discovered I was Earl and Cathy's nephew, her entire demeanor changed. She acted like I was a celebrity or an old friend. She got all flustered and made a big fuss over me. She called out to her husband, "Sam, this is Adam Hale, Earl and Cathy's nephew." Sam slowly walked towards us. He looked a lot like the old guy in Grant Wood's famous painting, with the pitchfork and wrinkled, stern face. He wore faded denim overalls, chewed on an old cigar and wore a serious expression.

He grasped my hand very firmly. "It's a pleasure to meet you, son. I'm Sam." "Hi. I'm Adam Hale. You know my Uncle Earl?"

"Everybody around here knows your uncle, son. After you're settled in, I'll tell you a little story about him." He paused about five seconds, then asked seriously, "Why are you stayin' here when you've got family in town?"

I didn't know quite what to say, so I said, "I want to surprise them later today or tomorrow. They don't know I'm here yet."

They both looked at me a little unsurely. Edna smiled politely and showed me to my room upstairs.

After a shower and a little nap, I went downstairs. Edna was cooking in the kitchen, so she suggested I join Sam on the porch.

I thought I'd try some down-home talk. "What kind of trees are those big ones around the house, Sam? They sure are beautiful."

"They're Ponderosa Pines," he answered proudly, like he created them himself. "My great-grandfather planted them over 100 years ago. People said they wouldn't live at this altitude, but there they are."

"I guess you've lived here your entire life then, huh?" I kind of liked this lazy, late afternoon, front porch talk.

"Born in that very room you're sleepin' in tonight. And six of our eight children were born right here, too."

I hope that's not the original bed still up there, I thought. "Wow. I bet you've seen a lot of changes around here through the years."

He looked at me as though he was trying to figure me out. "Sure have, lots of changes. My father owned one of the first cars in town. Everybody laughed at him, saying that a motorized carriage would never catch on. It was the noisiest darn thing you ever heard." I thought I detected a slight smile from his serious face as he mentioned the car.

"Sam, the first car? When were you born?"

"Nineteen-ten." He paused and spoke slowly. "I can still remember him drivin' it up this hill, all noisy and smoky. I was just a small boy then. I think I was feedin' the horses when I heard this awful racket comin' up the hill. There was Pa, behind the wheel of this slow-movin', smoky noisemaker." He chuckled a bit, caught himself, and then got serious again.

Sam seemed like an old-timer, but 105? I had no idea he was that old. Maybe he could shed some light on the strangeness of Southold Springs and my Uncle Earl. "I guess you were here when my uncle first moved to this town. It seems like a lot of people go to him. Does that seem odd to you?"

He looked at me a little strangely. "Odd? Your uncle changed our lives and the lives of lots of folks here. People go to him because he's a fine doctor and because he makes their lives better. Plain and simple."

I looked at him closely. His eyes were sharp, not dull and cloudy like most really old people I'd seen. It was hard for me to believe I was talking to a man more than 100 years old who could still hold an intelligent conversation. Now that I thought about it, he walked pretty well, too. Slow, but upright, with a good stride, not stooped over and hunchbacked.

"You want to hear a story about my daughter, Grace? She was my eighth child, born in 1969. All our other kids were strong and healthy, but Grace was sickly from birth. Doctors told us it was 'cause we had her when Edna was too old. Well, one night when Grace was about two months old, Edna heard a strange sound coming from her crib. She rushed to her, then quickly screamed out for me. Grace's little body wriggled in a twisted, spastic mass of rigid muscles. Her head moved back and forth like she was possessed by the devil himself. Her arms and legs twitched and flailed wildly. I tried to pick her up but couldn't. Her muscles were too wild and strong. After two or three minutes of this, her little body went limp. We weren't sure if she was breathin' or not, and had no idea what to do, so we called ol' Doc Johnson, who delivered her, but he didn't know what to do either. Doc stayed the night with us, then told us to get her to the big hospital in Denver in the morning.

"They ran so many tests on her little body. After three or four days in the hospital, they said she had epilepsy. They gave us some medicine for her, but it didn't do any good. She kept havin' more and more seizures. Sometimes she broke an arm or a leg when she had one real bad. Years went by. She never spoke a word, and never walked a step. She never even looked into our eyes. She always had this blank look on her face, staring straight out into space. And her seizures got more violent and more frequent. We took her to specialists all over the country. Nobody could help her. They told us to institutionalize her." Sam paused to chew on his cigar stub, and spit out a little tobacco over the rail of the porch.

"So here she was, seven and a half years old. No talkin', no walkin'. Nothin'. Just a body barely alive. Edna said she would never put her in one of those places, so we carried her around with us wherever we went. It was like her little body was alive, but nobody was home. And her seizures kept on gettin' worse. You could just see the life in her gettin' weaker and weaker all the time. After one really bad seizure, Doc Johnson told us that little Grace was goin' to die soon, so we better make preparations."

He got a little emotional, but continued.

"One day, a friend suggested we try this new doctor in town, a chiropractor. Doc Earl had only been in town a few months, so most of us never heard much about him. And to tell you the truth, we'd never even heard of a chiropractor back then, so we had no idea what he did. When we asked Doc Johnson about Doc Earl, he said that he was a quack. He also said that he wasn't a real doctor, he had no license, and we should stay away from him. But Edna insisted we talk to Doc Earl, so we did.

"Doc Earl had this little office in town – one room with one little table and a few chairs in it. He talked with us and asked lots of questions for quite some time. Then he said, 'Let's check Grace's spine.' He ran his fingers up and down Grace's little back. When he felt her upper neck, he asked us if we ever noticed this bone sticking out to the right. We said *yeah*, and we asked one of the doctors about it once, but he said it was nothin'. Doc Earl said that he was goin' to adjust that bone from right to left to take the pressure off little Grace's spinal cord. I looked at Edna. She looked back at me. We both shrugged our shoulders and said, 'OK'.

"Doc Earl placed his thumb on Grace's neck and pushed. 'Crack' went the bone, as loud as if someone busted a tree branch over his knee. The three of us went silent for a second or two. Edna thought that Doc Earl had just killed her youngest child, when suddenly, Grace turned her neck and looked up at Edna. Their eyes met. Grace then mumbled *Mommy*.

"All three of us stood there, stunned. None of us could talk for a solid minute. Then Edna started cryin' hysterically. I cried. Earl cried." Sam stopped to wipe a tear from his eye. "We took her home and little Grace never had another seizure. Less than a year later, she was in the first grade, a normal, healthy girl."

We sat in silence for a minute or two until Edna called us in for supper.

If you love a thing enough, it'll give up its secrets.
George Washington Carver

4

It was almost seven o'clock when I pulled into the large parking lot behind Uncle Earl's office in town. There were more than two dozen cars in the lot, and the office was just as busy. I was a bit nervous when I asked the woman at the front desk if Earl was in. She told me he was on his way downstairs. At that moment, Uncle Earl walked in and gave me a big, warm hug. "Would you look at you, Adam? Congratulations on graduating college and getting into med school."

"Thanks, Uncle Earl. It's good to see you. Where's Aunt Cathy?"

"Upstairs. I'm on my way to Oak Creek to give a talk. Run up and say hi, then hustle back down and you can take a ride with me if you've got the time."

I said *sure*, ran upstairs and said hello to my Aunt Cathy. When I told her I'd be around for the weekend, she said, "Alright, I'm glad we'll have some time together. But now, you go catch up to your uncle and have a safe trip. I'll make dinner for us all tomorrow night." She hugged and kissed me again and I walked downstairs.

I hopped in the passenger seat of Uncle Earl's Jeep, and we headed north to Oak Creek.

Uncle Earl smiled broadly, obviously very glad to see me. "How's everyone back east, Adam?"

"Fine. Mom and dad are well. Dad was planning on Mike going into practice with him, but Mike's thinking about emergency room medicine instead. Dad's disappointed, but now plans to wait for me to become a pediatrician to work with him and eventually take over his practice."

"Is that what *you* want, Adam?"

"Well, I guess so, but I'm not really sure. I like kids, but I also think about being a neurosurgeon sometimes. The brain always fascinated me." Uncle Earl smiled and said, "Me too."

We continued with the small talk for a while, and I felt safe in his company, so I just blurted out what was on my mind. "Why does my dad think you're crazy and dangerous? And why haven't you spoken to each other for the past 12 years?"

Uncle Earl smiled slightly. "I don't think your dad thinks I'm crazy. He just doesn't understand what I do."

"You mean chiropractics?"

"Chiroprac*tic*. There's no 's' on the end. Yes. I heard a lecture on chiropractic during my second year of medical school, and not only did it change my direction in life, but I began to speak out against some of the things your grandfather and father held quite dearly."

Dad's and Uncle Earl's father was a pediatrician, too. He died when I was a young boy, so I don't remember too much about him. Dad wanted my brother Mike and me to continue the family line of pediatricians.

I looked at his warm, blue eyes. He didn't look at all dangerous, but I had to ask, "Why would dad call you dangerous?"

He gave me a sad smile. "Medical propaganda. Your dad just happens to buy into it. For decades, medical schools taught their students that chiropractors were uneducated and unscientific cultists, and should be avoided."

I asked him about the day he adjusted my neck. "I never got to thank you for getting rid of my asthma. You left without saying goodbye. Thank you."

"You're welcome, Adam. I'm sorry, but when your dad returned to the summer house that day and heard that I had adjusted you, he was livid. He was angry with your mom for allowing it, but he was furious with me. I told him to get off his high horse and realize that there are other tools besides western medicine in this world. I said that if he was such a good doctor, why did his son suffer so? I guess that wasn't too bright on my part, because it just made him angrier. I left the house that evening." He let out a deep sigh. "The fact that a single chiropractic adjustment helped you after a dozen doctors had failed miserably was too strong a blow to the ego of someone as proud and intelligent as your dad."

I didn't know quite what to say. "Dad *was* glad that I had no more asthma, Uncle Earl." He smiled sadly again.

"You see, Adam, it's almost impossible for medicine to acknowledge the principles of chiropractic. If they acknowledged the fact that an adjustment reduced nerve interference and restored balance to a malfunctioning body, they would have to acknowledge the fact that it's wise for every person under every circumstance, *regardless* of the presence or absence of disease or symptoms, to have his or her spine checked regularly for vertebral subluxations, which are detrimental changes in the position, tension and mobility of the spine. You'll hear more about subluxation in a little while."

"But I thought medicine recognized chiropractic these days?"

He laughed. "Sure, as long as we don't rock their boat. Some members of the medical community say that chiropractors are okay for certain musculo-skeletal ailments, mostly low back pain. But the saddest thing is that many chiropractors jump for joy when they hear that. There are a large number of chiropractors that either reject, or are completely unaware of basic chiropractic philosophy, but they are chiropractors nonetheless. When a chiropractor's philosophy is weak or vague, his objective and practice is usually pain and symptom-oriented, and you don't often find children and asymptomatic people there. Sadly, this has contributed greatly to much of the confusion in our profession. The result is that the public hasn't a clue as to what chiropractic really is and how it can help people enjoy a far greater quality of life. To much of the public, we *crack* backs, massage, or use machines to ease back pain. When they hear of a 10-year-old going to a chiropractor for asthma, they think, *what in the world does a chiropractor have to do with asthma?* But it is this ignorance that often keeps people sick and dependent on medicine. No other profession in the world is so misunderstood. People know what dentists do. They know what accountants do. They know what architects do. But they don't know what chiropractors do. They *think* they know, but they really don't."

I asked, "Whose fault is that, Uncle Earl?"

"I believe it's a combination of things. In an attempt to be more scientific and avoid medical persecution, many chiropractors rejected the ideas of innate intelligence and subluxation and turned to a more musculo-skeletal approach and thereby became more therapeutic. In their minds, the lack of scientific research and evidence in chiropractic created an uncertain philosophy and a need to look elsewhere for acceptance. Many chiropractors simply didn't want to swim against the current of mainstream medical thinking. Also, a lot of chiropractors don't feel that the chiropractic adjustment is enough. They too, are more interested in pain and symptom relief. Sadly, most chiropractic colleges are not teaching chiropractic philosophy anymore. They are turning out graduates who don't see what Dr. B.J. Palmer, the man responsible for getting chiropractic out to the world, called the Big Idea, which is the profound simplicity of subluxation correction. They've worked hard and earned the degree of doctor of chiropractic, but they have no real understanding of chiropractic's great value to mankind. And so they set up an office and advertise that they treat low back pain, neck pain, shoulder pain, sciatica and headaches. They compete with medical doctors, emergency rooms, massage therapists, physical therapists and pain management clinics for all the people with back pain. How sad. In their hands, they hold a great gift for the better health and performance of mankind, and instead they toil each day trying to relieve backaches. And let's face it, Adam, what's the quickest way to get rid of pain?"

I thought for a moment and answered, "Take medicine."

Uncle Earl laughed and said, "Exactly. They won't improve your health or address the *cause* of your pain, but drugs can often alleviate pain quickly. Why chiropractors would want to compete with drugs is beyond me.

He continued. "Throughout chiropractic's history, there has been a great divide in our philosophy. And although there's a broad spectrum of chiropractic practices and philosophies, for decades the divisions have been labeled straights and mixers. I'm simplifying this a lot, but basically straight chiropractors locate, analyze and correct vertebral subluxations *by hand*, while mixers use various tools such as ice, heat, ultrasound, electric muscle and nerve stimulating devices, diathermy, nutrition, acupuncture, acupressure, exercise therapy, traction, decompression and dozens of other things. In my opinion, these tools are used by these chiropractors simply because, to them, the chiropractic adjustment is not enough. Their focus is on relief, and so they feel they have to *do* more to please the patient.

"When chiropractors utilize these various tools, the biggest problem is that it adds to the public's confusion about chiropractic. Even when someone else performs these services, if they're done in a chiropractic office, it's still confusing to the public. If you randomly asked 100 people what chiropractic is, you'll get 100 different answers, and 99 of them will likely be wrong.

"When it comes to chiropractic philosophy, the big split lies in objective. If a chiropractor's objective is to relieve low back pain, then he uses these various tools to get the patient feeling better as quickly as possible. To me, that's more like a form of manipulative medicine, and not chiropractic. And that's not to say there's anything wrong with trying to help your fellow man get out of pain. It's just not what B.J. Palmer and his father, D.D. Palmer, had in mind when they discovered and developed chiropractic. Chiropractic began with a deaf man's hearing being restored, and in its early history helped people with heart disease, cancer, diabetes, digestive disorders and mental illness. As medicine proceeded to dominate the health care landscape in the mid 20th century, chiropractic allowed itself to get pushed into a little corner of treating people with back and neck pain, shoulder pain and sciatica.

"Fortunately, there have always been a number of chiropractors that have adhered to the basic principles in chiropractic. They are the ones that see and adjust lots of kids and asymptomatic people. Why? Because chiropractic is *pro*active and not *re*active, and because these chiropractors understand that a little uncorrected subluxation is the beginning of spinal joint and disc degeneration, as well as the precursor to all kinds of mechanical, organic, glandular, neurological and immunological problems. Doesn't it make more sense to correct the subluxations in a young child *before* they become symptomatic? Isn't it foolish to wait until someone has a bulging disc and agonizing sciatica and *then* try to get them well?"

He took a deep breath and continued. "So, Adam, what about little Grace, who was severely autistic and epileptic for almost eight years until a chiropractic adjustment allowed her to become a normal, healthy girl? What about Billy, whose *alligator-skin* from head to toe, caused him to quit high school because the other kids teased him so badly? I adjusted his first cervical vertebra six times in two weeks and his skin cleared up. Completely. What about Joyce, whose kidneys functioned again after a series of adjustments?" His voice rose a bit. "What about all the really sick people in the world? Should they wait until they have back pain to see a chiropractor? Should all these kids with ear, sinus and upper respiratory infections, asthma, allergies, headaches and weakened immune systems be on all these horrible drugs for years, and have tubes put in their ears, and their tonsils cut out?"

"Do you treat all those things in your office, Uncle Earl?"

He swerved slightly to avoid a small animal. "I don't treat *any* disease or condition, Adam. I correct subluxations, period. I know it sounds simplistic, and it is. Vertebral subluxation is very real, and very devastating to the human body and mind, and as long as I'm alive, I'm going to teach people about it. They can put me in jail, call me a back-cracker or bone-crusher and that's okay. I know what I am and that what I do is right."

We traveled in silence for a while. "Tell me about the deaf man and how chiropractic began."

"In 1895, in Davenport, Iowa, a man named Daniel David Palmer, known as D.D., adjusted the spine of a deaf man, Harvey Lillard. Harvey regained his hearing and chiropractic was born. The word chiropractic, by the way, means *done by hand*. Well, I think Palmer thought he found a cure for deafness, and as he checked and adjusted the spines of many people during the following months and years, he found that it helped people with all different kinds of ailments and diseases. I believe he then thought he had found the cure for *all* diseases. Keep in mind – the philosophy had not yet been fully formed at this time. D.D. gradually developed the philosophy, but it wasn't until his son, B.J., took hold of it and spread the principle of specific subluxation correction to the world.

"B.J. toiled for decades to keep chiropractic a pure and distinct profession. He fought unbelievable odds. He persevered in spite of problems within the profession – those who abandoned the original principles – and also those outside the profession, primarily organized medicine that tried to eliminate chiropractic at every turn. He went years with very little sleep. He studied the human body possibly as deeply as anyone who has ever lived. He had the world's largest collection of human skeletons, and he studied each and every spine in great depth. He wrote volumes, lectured, and traveled throughout the world. He ran the Palmer College of Chiropractic, as well as a large clinic with chiropractors and medical doctors. He designed and used scientific equipment to validate the presence and damaging effects of subluxation, as well as the beneficial effects of correcting those subluxations.

"If you research B.J. Palmer, or ask people about him, you may hear words like *crazy* or *showman*. He certainly was different, but he wasn't crazy. And a showman? Yeah, he was a master. Chiropractic never would have survived without his showmanship, his dedication and his love and passion for this simple principle; that life is sweeter, that the human body and mind work better, and that *everyone* is better off with a subluxation-free spine and nervous system. He and his father had tapped into something very powerful, or had been given the gift and the responsibility to share this secret, known only by a few throughout the ages."

I asked, "Hadn't some form of manipulation been done before 1895?"

"Sure. An understanding of the importance of the spine has existed in various cultures throughout time. More than 2,000 years ago, Hippocrates, the father of medicine, stressed the importance of the spine and its relationship to health. These days, the understanding of the relationship between the structure of the spine and function of the nervous system is almost completely lost in medicine. Technology, drugs and surgery have taken over."

I was curious. "You said that medicine tried to eliminate chiropractic. What happened?"

"Chiropractic survived and grew because its principles are pure, logical and truthful, and also because it helped, and continues to help, many, many people." He paused to gather his thoughts. "After decades of negative propaganda and slander, with much of it directed at discrediting the founders, D.D. and B.J. Palmer, medicine tried to get rid of us by claiming that chiropractors were practicing medicine without a license. Chiropractic insisted that it was unique and distinct from medicine, and won in the courts. As you know, medicine is basically the diagnosis and treatment of disease. Its objective for thousands of years has been to treat and conquer disease. Chiropractic's objective is *not* the treatment of disease, but the location, analysis and correction of vertebral subluxation. Its goal is to improve the function of the human body and mind as a whole by improving the integrity of the central nervous system. In this regard, chiropractic is unique. It is not an *alternative* to medicine. It is not a *substitute* for medicine. I would never tell someone to get adjusted *instead of* seeking medical or any other care. I simply say get adjusted to improve the integrity of your nervous system, which in turn improves the function of your body and mind, which improves your overall quality of life. You know what happens with a healthier functioning body and mind? You need less medical care."

After a few minutes of silence, Uncle Earl spoke again. "Sadly, chiropractic lost its leadership after B.J. Palmer's death in 1961. Since then, chiropractors have taken the profession in various directions. Many have chosen a therapeutic, back pain/treatment model, which has greatly contributed to the large scale confusion within the profession, and consequently, in the public's eye. I cannot speak for the entire chiropractic community, but it is important that the world understands the beauty and simplicity of the chiropractic principles you're about to learn."

We cruised down a huge mountain into Oak Creek. Uncle Earl made a left turn and we pulled into a large, crowded parking lot adjacent to a square, brick American Legion Hall.

Chiropractic is specific or it's nothing.

B.J. Palmer

5

From the trunk of his car, Uncle Earl grabbed a large blue duffel bag. I offered to carry it for him, but he smiled and said, "No thanks. But you could carry this for me." He handed me two pieces of what looked like a wooden and metal coat rack.

Inside the clean but musty-smelling building were about a 100 people ranging in ages from their early 20s to some in their 70s and 80s. Uncle Earl led us to seats in the front row. In front of us was an old wooden table on a small stage. On the table were a microphone, a glass and a pitcher of water. For about 15 minutes, while 30 or more people came in and sat, I watched my uncle make small talk with a few people. He introduced me to Mayor Quinn, a short, stout, bald man, wearing a wrinkled, brown corduroy suit and a crooked, but friendly smile. Mayor Quinn shook my hand and welcomed me to Oak Creek. He clipped a small microphone to Uncle Earl's shirt and introduced him before my uncle spoke.

"Thank you Mayor Quinn, and thank you Oak Creek for having me here tonight. My name is Dr. Earl Hale, and I am a chiropractor. Tonight I'm going to teach you a little bit about life, health and the human body, specifically regarding a certain principle that I believe will help you live better lives. The principle I'm going to share with you incorporates some new terms, which I hope to make clear and understandable. These are *organization, intelligence, subluxation* and *adjustment*. I ask you to open your minds and hearts a bit, think, and challenge my logic, my thoughts and words if you will. I'll be happy to answer questions later."

Earl sipped some water and smiled at his audience. "How many people here believe in God or some higher power?" With a little commotion, about 80 percent of the group raised their hands.

"No, I'm not going to preach or talk religion. I just want to get a little feel for the group. We're going to start from the beginning, so the first topic I'd like to discuss is the miracle of birth." From his duffel bag, he took out a life-sized doll, which looked very much like a real baby. He laid it gently on the table.

"Basically, there are two ways of looking at life – random or organized. We in chiropractic choose to see life as organized and purposeful. Please let me explain. Two tiny half-cells, the sperm and the egg, unite to form one whole cell, and then it slowly divides. Two cells, four, eight, 16, 32, 64. You get the idea. A couple of weeks down the road and we have a small blob of cells, kind of like a little mulberry or raspberry. It certainly doesn't look like a little person yet." A few people chuckled. "*Something* causes this little blob of cells to change. Some *power,* some *intelligence* or *force* is at work here. In order to form a baby, we need a lot of different cells and tissues to form. And very importantly, we need them to be *organized.* Organization is the first key concept here, and at the very heart of chiropractic is the idea that organization implies intelligence. We state that when something is organized, *something* had to cause that organization. Some kind of force or intelligence. You don't want your baby's heart in his arm, or his lungs where his kidneys should be, right?

"Let me give you an example of organization and intelligence; let's take a wristwatch apart and put its 100-plus pieces in your hands. Now toss them into the air and let them land on the ground. Will they come together on the ground and form a fully functional watch again? Of course not. Suppose we do it a thousand times? Will it be a watch again? A million times?"

"No", a few answered with a laugh.

"It wouldn't happen if we did it ten million times because a wristwatch must be put together intelligently and purposefully in order to function properly. We in chiropractic see the human body as organized and intelligent. The information within the DNA of living organisms is more vibration, or energy than it is matter, and yet that energy inside a single cell has the power and intelligence to divide into trillions upon trillions of cells, all harmoniously organized to become you and me – breathing, loving, thinking, feeling, brilliant people. How's that for intelligence?"

The audience laughed again.

"OK, back to the blob of cells. First a dark spot shows up in the blob, followed by a dark line extending from the dark spot. The cells continue to divide and change, eventually forming bones, muscles, blood vessels, nerves, organs, glands, arms and legs. Wow!" He paused for effect, and then added slowly, "Nine months go by and *voila*, a beautiful, bouncing baby boy or girl. Hopefully. Provided nothing *interfered* with the process. There's our miracle. All agreed?" He held up the doll baby. "Pretty amazing, huh? And it happens billions and billions of times every day. Not just humans, but bugs and lizards and mice and squirrels and birds and fish and cats and dogs and elephants. This is the great miracle of life covered in about four minutes." More chuckles from the crowd.

"Although reproduction is a function of all living things, I'm going to keep the focus on vertebrates, animals with spines, and most importantly, humans. Everybody with me so far? Good." In a joking, teacher-like tone, he added, "We're going to go back to that little blob of cells in a while, so I hope you were all paying attention.

"What makes a living body different from an inanimate thing, such as this table or microphone?" Without waiting for a reply, he said, "What it does and how it behaves. How it *expresses* itself. In other words, a living thing changes itself, changes its physiology to survive. A living thing is capable of *re-organizing* itself to perpetuate its existence. If you cut your finger, the tissues will reorganize themselves to seal the wound, form a scab and heal. But if I cut the finger of this doll, it doesn't change. We can examine the doll five years from now and that cut will still be there. It doesn't have the innate ability to change, to reorganize itself and heal."

He paused, took a drink of water and held out the glass. "If I drop this glass on the floor, it will break into many pieces. It will no longer be a useful glass. And unless some kind of intelligence, like a person, glues the pieces back together, it could never be a glass again. Like the watch, it does not have the capability, the *intelligence* within itself to return to the form of a useful glass."

He laid the glass back down and continued. "But if *I* fall on the floor here and break my leg, what happens?" Someone in the audience yelled out "You sue us!" and everyone laughed. Uncle Earl laughed too, and said, "Oh, there's a lawyer in every crowd. No, I don't have to sue you. My body knows how to re-organize itself and repair the broken bone. Herein lies a great advantage of being alive. Living beings contain an inborn or *innate* intelligence, and it is this same intelligence that causes the sperm and egg cell to unite and divide, then differentiate, or create different cells and tissues. Within the microscopic DNA of those two cells is all the information to create that little miracle. One cell becomes trillions and trillions of cells, all different, but all united to allow us to breathe, think, see and live. I'd say that's intelligent." He looked a little more serious and spoke slower. "Now, do you think that when we're born, this intelligence leaves us? No, it doesn't. The miracle, the magic, is always in us. Whether we're two days old, two years old, or 92 years old, this innate intelligence is running our bodies, healing, repairing and replacing cells every minute of our lives.

"So whether you come from a religious perspective or a scientific one, I think it's safe to acknowledge that there is *some* kind of wisdom, *some* form of intelligence running our bodies all our lives. We don't have to think about healing a simple cut on our hand or digesting the corn flakes we had for breakfast. The body knows *exactly* what to do. Miraculous." He paused, then added, "Albert Einstein helped discover the atom bomb because he understood the enormous power within the atom. Similarly, we in chiropractic understand the great power residing in every atom and fiber of living organisms. We call it *innate intelligence*, and we state that it uses the nervous system to express itself. I don't think it matters much what you call this inborn intelligence; God, spirit, life force, nature or science. What matters is that you recognize it as a vital part of who you are.

"In chiropractic, we don't try to control or manipulate this innate intelligence. Instead, our objective is to *allow* it to express itself fully and unrestricted. After all, it *did* know how to create the entire body. We know that although this intelligence exists within every part of our being, the body needs a properly functioning nervous system in order to express it. How do we know that? Simple. When the nerve supply to any part of the body is cut off, that body part will not work properly or at all. Sometimes, that body part will simply die. The intelligence is within every cell, but it needs the nervous system to allow its proper function and expression.

"OK, again we're back to the little blob of cells on their way to becoming a fully-formed, fully-functional human being. Remember the little dark spot with the dark line extending from it? The very first *different* thing to show up in the blob of cells? They are the beginning of the brain and spinal cord. They grow and expand, form branches, and *then* organs and glands, arms and legs begin to develop from the growing nervous system. Like apples that can only grow *after* the tree is created, the rest of the body develops around the brain and spinal cord. Why? Because the brain and spinal cord connect all parts of the body to each other. The extremely intricate nervous system ties the whole thing together, offering lines of communication among all cells and tissues.

"The body is made up of cells. Groups of similar cells are called tissues, such as muscle, bone and connective tissue. When different tissues come together with a common purpose, that's called an organ. Think of an organ as a group of tissues *organ-* ized to perform a specific task or function. A kidney is an organ designed to filter the blood. A lung is an organ designed to extract oxygen from the air. I don't want to teach anatomy here. I want you to get an idea of the whole body, the whole picture, and what makes it all tick. I want you to get a feel for the magnificence of the great force that has put this little newborn baby's body together."

An old man with a walker in front of him, a few seats to my right, suddenly asked, somewhat annoyed, "What does this stuff have to do with healing? I've got a lot of problems and I don't know why you're talking about birth and cells and stuff."

Uncle Earl walked toward the man and spoke very slowly and gently. "How we think and how we feel has a great effect on how we heal. I'm not quite sure what you were expecting tonight, but I assure you that what I offer is genuine and can help you greatly. If you are thinking I've got some magic to work instantly on you, I don't. Part of the purpose of this portion of the talk is to get you to look *inside* yourself; to see the real magic and power that's within you. I want you to understand that healing comes from within. I've found that unless I present some background and understanding of these concepts, many people don't get the big idea that I'm trying to share with you. And, I *am* going to share a big idea with you."

He walked towards the center of the stage. "I'm not trying to change your way of thinking. I'm trying to add to it. And I'm pretty sure that what I have to say is new and different to most of you, so please bear with me. Thank you for your question, sir.

"What I'm leading into is an understanding of the importance of your spines and nervous systems. Because of their complexity, their relationship is poorly understood by most, and sadly, they are two of the most neglected parts of the body. In fact, most people take better care of their teeth, their hair and their nails, all things you can actually live without. So in order to answer this gentleman's question, let's get right to the heart of the matter." He raised his voice a little and enunciated each word slowly, "Your brain and spinal cord are the most important parts of your entire body and affect every single cell, organ, gland and tissue in your body. Everything!" He took a few deep breaths and gathered his thoughts.

"Mother Nature, in her wisdom, protects two parts of the human body by surrounding them with bone. Do you know what those two parts are?" A few people called out, *the brain*. "Right. The brain *and* the spinal cord. The brain is surrounded and well protected by the bones of the skull, and the bones of the spine, called vertebrae, surround the spinal cord. There are 24 of these bones, and they line up, one on top of the other like a stack of donuts, forming the spinal column." He reached into his large, blue bag and pulled out a model of a spine. He held it up and said, "This is a plastic model of what your spine looks like. Please pass this around and get a little feel for it. Feel the movement of each bone and its relationship to its neighbors." He handed it to the old man to my right. "Go ahead. Bend it. Twist it. This is your spine, and running down the middle of it is an extension of your brain called the spinal cord. Also, notice the spinal nerves that exit from in between the vertebrae. They go to and from *everything* in your body.

"Science tells us that every cell in the body has nerve fibers connected to it. *Every* cell. Did you ever get a tiny splinter in your finger, like a small hair from a cactus? It hurts. Why? Because it's causing a few nerve fibers to send pain messages to the brain. As soon as that little splinter comes out, it feels better. Science also tells us that there are trillions of brain cells and trillions of fibers running down the spinal cord. Put simply, the brain can send and receive a lot of information. And it does most of this without the slightest awareness on our part."

A man to my right handed me the plastic spine. I noticed that the bones go from smaller ones in the neck to thicker ones in the low back. I twisted it, thinking that, although I knew what the spine looked like from basic anatomy classes, I never really thought about its relation to the brain and organs and glands of the body. I passed it to the middle-aged woman on my left.

Uncle Earl continued, "Please understand, more than 99 percent of everything your body does is done automatically. Unconsciously. Without your help or awareness. You don't have to think about regulating blood pressure, body temperature, heart rate, digestion, respiration, blood sugar levels, the constriction and dilation of your pupils, hormone production, cellular repair and replacement, and thousands of other things that go on inside your body. If you had to consciously accomplish everything your body did innately, you'd die before you were a minute old.

"Before I continue talking about the structure of the spine, I want to wait until you all get a chance to see and feel the plastic model. In the meantime, let's talk about body chemistry. The cells, organs and glands of your body produce thousands of chemicals every minute of your life. And these cells, organs and glands know exactly *when* to produce the proper chemical, and exactly *how much* of the chemical that's needed by the body at that moment. For example, when you take a bite of that tuna fish sandwich you had for lunch, there are cells in your salivary glands that produce an enzyme called ptyalin, which helps break down the starch in the bread. At the same time, cells in your stomach, called parietal cells, produce hydrochloric acid to break down the protein in the tuna.

Real hydrochloric acid. And if there's mayonnaise in your sandwich, your gall bladder will squirt out just the right amount of bile to help break down the fats in the mayo. This is just a small part of what happens when you take a bite of that sandwich. The wisdom of your body knows how to take this sandwich and have it become part of your body. Wow!" He paused to let this sink in.

"Wait a second. How does the stomach know *when* to produce the hydrochloric acid? And how do the salivary glands and gall bladder know *when* and *how much* to produce of their chemicals? Good questions. How? Because of the nervous system. The brain and spinal cord direct all the cells, organs and glands into action, into production and secretion. How well your body works depends on how well the cells produce the quantity and quality of the chemicals needed. And it's not just digestion. It's *everything*. To fall asleep your body must produce chemicals. To wake up it must produce chemicals. To run, to think, to have sex, to breathe. All by changing your body chemistry. Your chemistry determines how well your body and mind perform. How your body and mind perform determines how well your life works."

His voice rose in intensity. "Let's take this a step further, and this is a basic principle unfamiliar to most doctors and laypeople alike; the chemistry of your body is determined by the electrical system of your body. Yes, I'm aware that the nervous system is chemical as well as electrical, but I want to keep this as simple as possible. In other words, your nervous system, the electrical system of the body, determines how well the organs and glands of your body work. This is why bones protect your brain and spinal cord – they are essential to every function of your body and mind, and every aspect of your life!"

He reached into his blue duffel bag and pulled out a life-size, clear plastic head and torso. Inside it I could see a heart, lungs, stomach, intestines and other organs. He also grabbed an extension cord and asked me to plug it in for him. I found an outlet and did so, and the organs inside the clear body glowed with different colored lights. Uncle Earl hung the glowing torso on the metal and wooden stand so everyone could see it.

"So, have most of you seen the model of the spine yet?" A few rows of people in the back had not yet seen it. "As I said before, most of us know that the brain is well-protected inside the skull bones, but most are unaware of the way the spinal cord and spinal nerves are protected by the bones of the spine. Notice how the joints of the vertebrae meet each other. Notice the discs between the vertebrae, which act as cushions or shock absorbers. And keep in mind that there are lots of muscles and ligaments holding it all together as well." He pointed to his clear plastic torso, and turned it around so we could see its back. "My clear man here has no vertebrae in his back. Instead, I've installed a series of dimmer switches like the ones in your dining rooms. The wires from each dimmer switch represent the spinal nerve roots that exit from in between each vertebra.

"To know how important your nervous system is to all parts of the body, let's cut a nerve and see what happens. Guess what happens if we clip the nerves going to your lungs? They don't work. You die. How about your kidneys? Same thing. Your pancreas? Your thyroid? Your fingers? All the same. Well, you don't die if we cut the nerve to one of your fingers, but the finger won't work." He unplugged the extension cord from the back of the clear torso and all the lights inside it went out. "You see what I'm getting at, don't you? When I cut off the electrical supply, the lights go out, right? That's called death, by the way." He plugged it back in to a few nervous chuckles.

"The next concept I'm going to teach you today is the most important aspect of chiropractic – the vertebral subluxation. A subluxation is a change in the position or mobility of one or more of these vertebrae. It is a spinal injury that has not healed properly. It is a sprain of a spinal joint, similar to a sprain of an ankle or any other joint, with one big exception; it *alters nerve function*. It changes the way your nervous system works."

He took a deep breath and continued. "The bones of the skull protect the delicate tissues of the brain very well. They only move very, very slightly. But the bones of the spine? They move a lot!" Uncle Earl did a corny little dance on the stage to demonstrate the movement of the spine. "They are held together by many joints, which allow us to bend and twist and jump and dance. Do you know how many joints there are in your spine from the base of your skull to your tailbone? 101. One hundred and one joints allow great movement, but they are also potential sites for injury. Compare that to other parts of your body. How many hip joints do we have?" A few people yelled out, *two*. "Right. And knee joints? Also two. Nothing in your body is similar to your spine. Only the hands and feet come close to having 101 joints, but they too are nothing like the spine. Your spine is unique."

A young boy returned the plastic spine and Uncle Earl thanked him. "Occasionally someone asks me how a spine is injured. I usually answer that question with further questions. Have you ever watched a playful two-year-old doing somersaults or a child learning to walk or ride a two-wheeled bike or a skateboard? Have you ever seen the collisions on a soccer or football field? Can you imagine the impact to a spine during a car accident? Science has proven that necks are often injured during the birth process, sometimes to the point of killing the newborn baby. The point is that our spines take a beating throughout our lives. They are injured time and time again, and although we heal from many of these injuries, sometimes we don't. The vertebrae get stuck, and the injured joint loses its range of motion and causes a gradual breakdown, not only mechanically, but neurologically as well. If you want to see the effects of uncorrected vertebral subluxations, just look at some old timers – hunchbacked, bent over and rigid. It's very obvious sometimes, and it almost always manifests as flexion. You don't see these old people in extension, with their heads held high and chests out. Instead, their heads bend forward until they need a cane, then a walker, and then a wheelchair. Flexion brings you closer to death.

"There are many causes of vertebral subluxation, but the most common are physical or mechanical traumas, chemical stresses, and emotional and mental stresses. These can all have a very negative impact on the spine and nervous system. How many of you here have watched videos on YouTube?" About two-thirds of the audience raised their hands. "Ever seen some that show kids falling off their skateboards or roller blades? Ouch! Subluxation. Ever seen a baby learning to walk? Step – fall, step – fall, step – fall. Subluxation. We've already mentioned traumatic birth. Many of us enter this world very violently, and we often start our lives with severely subluxated spines, which means we are literally weakened from birth.

"How many of you have ever slipped on the ice or been in a car accident? Subluxation. How many played contact sports? Subluxation. How many sit for long hours driving, or at the computer or television? Subluxation. And these are just the physical causes of spinal injuries. Chemical, emotional and mental stresses can also change the position and tension of the spine and spinal cord causing subluxation. Anger, jealousy, resentment, anxiety and fear all increase tension in the spine, nervous system and body. The human spine manifests the effects of life's traumas and stresses. It's designed to endure a lot, but if you look at the posture and tone of people, detrimental changes to the spine are often quite obvious. But the key is to address them *before* they become obvious. That's one of chiropractic's great benefits."

He pulled the clear plastic torso closer to the audience. "A vertebral subluxation does not *completely* cut off the nerve supply to organs, glands, muscles or blood vessels. It's more like a dimmer switch. It blocks *some* of the energy feeding the organ or gland." He turned one of the dimmer switches in the back of his clear model and the light within the lungs dimmed. "Can everyone see clearly what happens when I turn this little knob?" A few people murmured *yes*. "If you'd like to come up closer, you're welcome to."

He turned down the lights on a few more organs and glands. "This is what a subluxation does to your body. It diminishes it. And when you diminish the function of even one little organ or gland, or *any* part for that matter, you diminish the whole body." He turned the lights on fully. "Here's another question for you. When I dim the light, oh, let's say to the lungs, for example…" He turned down a switch in the upper back and the bronchi and lungs dimmed. "Is the problem in the lungs?" He paused a moment. "It *appears* to be a problem in the lungs, doesn't it? Look, they're weak." The audience stirred a bit. "No, the problem is actually back here." He pointed to the switch in the upper back. "And don't think this isn't real. There has been scientific research that has demonstrated clearly the relationship between upper thoracic spinal changes and lung function. So, does this person need lung medication? Do you think that's the best thing for him? And no, I'm not saying that adjustments to the spine are a substitute or alternative for medical care, I just want you to *very clearly see* the relationship between the spine and the organs and glands of the body.

"Every organ and gland, muscle and tissue in the body has a specific nerve supply going to it. The major nerve pathways to the stomach are from the level of the sixth and seventh dorsal, right between your shoulder blades. Medical doctors treat the stomach when very often the problem is not in the stomach, but in the nerve supply *to the stomach*. You can treat and control the symptoms of asthma with drugs, but until you get the nerve supply to the bronchi and lungs working properly, you'll always have asthma. More often than not, asthma is *not* a bronchial or lung problem. It's a *neuro-logical* problem. And so it is often with gastritis, heartburn, irritable bowel syndrome, colitis, Crohn's Disease, kidney disease, uterine and ovarian problems, and just about anything else you can think of. It *appears* that the organ or gland is the problem, but it isn't. The real problem is in the nerve supply, and when that nerve supply is altered by vertebral subluxation, the organ or gland suffers and mal-functions. Of course, there are other factors with all sicknesses and diseases, but the wise thing to do is make sure the nervous system is working properly – first. Sadly, people endure a lifetime of treating a weak organ or gland with drugs and surgery, while the chiroprac-tor, the expert at removing interference in the nervous system, isn't even considered. The central nervous system, the major system of the entire body, is completely ignored by doctor after doctor."

He turned the lights on brightly again, then reached towards the back of the model's head. "A subluxation present anywhere in the spine has the potential to weaken the entire nervous system, but this is especially true of the upper cervical vertebrae where the spinal cord exits the brain." He turned an upper dimmer switch and all the organs and glands darkened. "Subluxations do this to your body. How do want your life to be, like *this*?" He pointed to the dimly lit body. Then he turned the lights on brightly. "Or like *this*?"

Uncle Earl paused, looked for a few flickers of recognition in the crowd and continued. "Chiropractic is about checking the spine from birth to make sure the power is fully turned on. A vertebral subluxation is a bad thing. It diminishes and weakens your body, your mind, and your life.

"The final concept I would like you to understand this eve-ning is the chiropractic adjustment. It's not a treatment. It's not a therapy. It's an *adjustment*, a freeing process. It is the application of a specific and intelligent force to reduce or correct a vertebral subluxation, thus allowing the central nervous system to work the way it's supposed to work.

"Let's say a baby girl has had a mildly traumatic birth, leaving her first cervical vertebra subluxated." He pointed to his neck, just below the ear. "It's causing significant weakness to her nervous and immune systems, and by the time she's a year old, she's had multiple ear infections, strep throat, and colic. She doesn't sleep through the night, so neither does mom or dad. Like most parents, they take her repeatedly to the pediatrician, who prescribes antibiotics and suppositories. Do the antibiotics make her stronger?" He paused and shook his head. "No, they don't. In fact, they weaken her. Do the suppositories make her stomach and intestines work better? No. So what should we do with this little girl and her weakened body? Leave her alone and see what happens? Wait until she has chronic tonsillitis or Crohn's Disease? Hope she *outgrows* these things? What should be done about that little bone in her neck irritating the spinal cord and spinal nerve roots? About that little subluxation that's diminishing her brain's ability to function?

"I think the logical, common sense thing to do would be to adjust that bone back into place. Sound reasonable? Sure it does. It's so simple and obvious, and yet the vast majority of pediatricians and parents don't know it. Sadly, no one has ever taught them about this intricate and powerful relationship between structure and function in the human body.

"Now please don't get me wrong. I'm not saying that the subluxation is the cause of *all* ear infections, sore throats or colic, but I *am* saying that logic dictates that when a child, or anyone for that matter, is sick or weakened in any way, the *very first thing* that should be examined is the nerve supply. After all, the central nervous system controls and coordinates every structure and function in the human body. But as it has for centuries, medicine still puts most of its attention on blood and its chemistry rather than nerves. And although the damage done to nerve roots from spinal injuries has been scientifically documented for decades, this is rarely in the medical person's thought processes when it comes to sickness and disease." He paused and stretched a bit.

"Now here are just a couple of key points regarding vertebral subluxation. One – you don't know when you're subluxated. I've been a chiropractor for more than 40 years, and *I* don't know when I'm subluxated. Subluxations don't always cause pain, especially initially, so ideally, it would be great if we had a big red light on our foreheads that lit up when we were subluxated. Then we'd know exactly when we needed to be adjusted. But we don't. So, when is the best time to get your spine checked and adjusted? When you're subluxated! How do you know if you're subluxated? You don't. Only a skilled chiropractor can tell you. This is why I recommend that everyone get their spines checked regularly by a chiropractor whose sole purpose is to locate, analyze and correct vertebral subluxations. And by regularly, I mean once a week or once every two weeks. Current research tells us that subluxated, sprained joints can cause permanent and irreversible damage – their words, not mine – within 10 to 14 days. So what does that mean? If your child is subluxated at birth, or from a fall at age two, and is now 10 years old, there's a lot of work that needs to be done to turn that child's life around. It may take months to correct, but it's always worth it when you understand the devastating effects of subluxation. Everyone deserves to go through life free from vertebral subluxation."

He took a big drink of water, smiled and said, "Thank you all so much for coming out tonight. I'll leave you with a little homework. *Observe* the spines and the tone and posture of people around you. Be polite. Don't stare, but observe with a keen eye. Look at your children. Look at your parents and grandparents. Look at your own spine. Do you move with ease and grace, or are you stiff and restricted? Does your neck turn to both sides equally and easily?" He paused and continued, "I wish you well on your journey towards better health and a richer life, and I recommend chiropractic care for every single person on earth because it's simple, logical and powerful, and it works every time. When a subluxation is reduced, even slightly, your central nervous system works better and your health and life are better. Good night and safe home."

A woman a few rows behind me waved her hand and abruptly asked, "Why'd you ask us if we believe in God at the start of your talk? What does that have to do with all you said?"

Uncle Earl smiled kindly at the woman and said, "Great question. People today, due to an amazingly powerful marketing campaign for the past 50 years or so, have come to put a lot of *faith* in medicine. Our religions teach us to have faith in God, but regarding our bodies, *our temples*, we've been taught in recent history to trust less in God or nature and more in man-made pharmaceuticals. If you've watched the news or read anything in the last few decades, you know about the many dangers of modern drugs. Chemistry in the human body is not a true science, but rather an ongoing history of trial and error experiments. Some drugs help and save lives, while others harm and kill people. My goal is to remind people of the great power, the wonderful intelligence that resides within each and every one of us. So I'm not suggesting we give up our faith in medicine, but I *am* suggesting we learn to put *some* faith and trust in the power that created our amazing body from those two little half-cells I spoke about earlier. Chiropractic's job is to allow the full and healthy expression of that innate intelligence by the correction of vertebral subluxations. There are many chiropractors like me who happen to place a very high degree of trust in that innate intelligence. I hope that answers your question. Thank you again, and good night."

The crowd clapped for awhile, and I watched as a dozen or so people came up front to talk with Uncle Earl. He patiently answered all their questions and then asked me to help him pack up.

One of the first duties of the physician is to educate the masses not to take medicine.

Sir William Osler

6

We drove in silence for a few minutes, but two questions gnawed at me. "Uncle Earl, a little while ago you said that chiropractic *always* works. That sounds a bit bold, to say the least."

Uncle Earl chuckled. "Adam, *every* chiropractic adjustment that corrects or reduces a subluxation, even the slightest bit, improves that person's spine and nervous system and makes his or her life better. Unfortunately, you and the rest of the western world have been taught to think in terms of symptoms only. Every adjustment does *not* make one feel better. An adjustment doesn't always magically remove symptoms immediately. It's not supposed to, although it does happen sometimes. Remember the purpose of a chiropractic adjustment?"

"To correct vertebral subluxation."

"Very good, Adam. You *are* paying attention." We both laughed at his sarcasm. "The big problem is that we're conditioned to think of health care as the treatment of symptoms. The majority of medicines, both over-the-counter and prescription, are directed at symptom relief. From headaches to athlete's foot, there are thousands of drugs designed to relieve symptoms, but very few that actually improve the health of the individual. The United States represents about 5 percent of the world's population, yet we take more than 80 percent of the painkillers in the world. Does that sound healthy to you? We consume huge percentages of the world's muscle relaxants, anti-inflammatory drugs, antidepressants and many other drugs, too. We are a drug-addicted culture. Millions rely on drugs for just about everything, and as far as I'm concerned, a drug is a drug is a drug."

"What do you mean by that?" I asked.

"I mean that every drug in the world is designed to do one of two things – change the way we feel or change the way we function. And the vast majority of drugs taken to change the way we feel simply diminish our ability *to* feel. Aches, pains, spasms, anxiety, depression. It doesn't matter what kind of pain or discomfort you have or where it is in your body or mind, there's a drug to make you feel better. Throughout the past 50 years or so, we've been taught, actually brainwashed, that drugs are good for us and that drugs contribute to a healthier society, but this is simply a lie. The World Health Organization ranks the U.S. somewhere around 38th in health. Pathetic. The misuse, overuse and abuse of drugs in our culture are actually making us sicker, weaker and more drug-dependent. I agree with physician Oliver Wendell Holmes' statement, *I firmly believe that if the whole materia medica, as now used, could be sunk to the bottom of the sea, it would be better for mankind – and all the worse for the fishes.*"

I laughed and changed the subject with my second question. "Uncle Earl, that story I heard from old Sam Sprague about his daughter sounded really ridiculous. How true is it?"

"It's true, Adam. Grace's life changed dramatically with one adjustment. These things happen in chiropractic offices around the world, although they're usually not this extreme or dramatic. This is what changed Southold Springs and my practice overnight. Everyone knew the Sprague family and Grace's condition, so that one adjustment grabbed the attention of the entire community. Actually, I consider myself very lucky to have that happen in my first year of practice in Colorado. It opened my eyes to the great power within the chiropractic adjustment, but it also gave me a lot of attention from the local family medical doctor, Doc Johnson."

I interrupted him. "I heard that he didn't like you, and that he tried to have you arrested. Is that true?"

"Didn't like me? He despised me. He was not only the local GP, but obstetrician and pediatrician as well. As more children came to me to get adjusted, their visits to him were noticeably less frequent. I remember one young boy about 10 or 11 years old. Even though Doc Johnson had been treating him for asthma and severe headaches for more than five years, this poor little boy's visits to the emergency room were more frequent, and he was slowly becoming more disabled. He couldn't play outside with other kids, couldn't participate in gym class, and couldn't even run up a flight of stairs without wheezing heavily. Well, after a few adjustments, the little guy never had an asthma attack or a headache again and never took his medicine again. This didn't sit too well with Dr. Johnson. You'd think he'd be happy for the little boy, but he was furious instead, kind of like your dad was when I adjusted you. Well, Doc Johnson would see me in public and call me a fraud and a charlatan. He'd do anything he could to embarrass or humiliate me. He told his patients that I was dangerous. He erroneously thought that I had told the boy not to take his medicine any more, something I would never do. That's when he tried to have me arrested for practicing medicine without a license.

"I asked Dr. Johnson if I could sit down with him, buy him lunch and teach him about what I do. He said he would never talk to me, let alone have a meal with me. I told him that we were both doing the same thing, trying to help people heal and live healthier lives. He got so angry when I said that I thought he would explode. He said that he was a man of science and that he could not consort with a cultist who was a non-medical quack." Uncle Earl smiled and stroked his beard. "As you can guess, we never became pals."

I laughed at his joke and said, "It doesn't make sense. Why would a doctor do that when you were obviously helping people?"

"Ignorance, fear, ego, power, loss of control – take your pick. And don't think it was just because it was the 1970s. Similar things still go on today in some cities and towns. In 1987, there was a landmark case – Wilk vs. AMA – that found the AMA guilty of conspiring to destroy chiropractic. Medicine finally removed the statement from their bylaws that strictly forbade medical doctors to consort with chiropractors.

"Chiropractic is a threat to the mechanistic, allopathic medical model. Of course many chiropractors these days try to be more like medical doctors, and many medical doctors seem to think chiropractors are okay *as long as we know our place*. Which means, as long as we chiropractors treat only low back pain and other *non-neurological* musculo-skeletal disorders." He frowned and shook his head. "Of course, to a principled chiropractor like me, *everything* we do is neurological. We correct subluxations, which are neurological as well as mechanical lesions."

He added sarcastically, "Yeah, we chiropractors are accepted now by medicine. Hallelujah!" His voice rose. "Some chiroprac*tors* are accepted, but chiroprac*tic* continues to be completely misunderstood by organized medicine and the public. Medicine would have to change its entire philosophy to accept chiroprac*tic*. And that doesn't seem likely to happen."

I interrupted, "You emphasize the syllables *tic* and *tor*. What do you mean by that?"

"I mean that chiroprac*tic* is a philosophy as well as a science and art, and that it has definite principles and objectives. Because chiroprac*tors* do so many different things in their offices, most people haven't a clue as to what chiroprac*tic's* philosophy and purpose are. When I say chiroprac*tic*, I mean the science, philosophy and art of the location and correction of vertebral subluxations.

"In most towns and cities throughout the country, you'll find a chiropractor who performs physical therapy, another who does nutritional counseling, another who practices acupuncture, and another who does foot reflexology and aromatherapy." Again his voice rose. "How in the world can we expect anyone to understand chiroprac*tic* when the chiroprac*tors* themselves don't have a uniform philosophy?" He paused a moment and added, "And I'm not saying there's anything wrong with any of these other things that chiropractors do. I just think it creates way too much confusion about chiroprac*tic*."

"Why do they choose to do all these other things then?" I asked.

"As I said before, many chiropractors are caught up in the medical model which is about pain and symptom relief, and so they reject the idea of subluxation correction and focus on whatever they can do to relieve pain."

"Do chiropractors take x-rays to find the subluxations?" I asked.

"Some do, but I don't believe you can measure a subluxation on an x-ray. You can see a misalignment on an x-ray, but that's not necessarily a subluxation. It may well be a compensation or adaptation. A subluxation is a dynamic change in an individual's spine and nervous system. This is why I often use the obvious example of an 80-year-old man or woman with a grossly distorted spine. You see them all over the world. Some of them are so distorted it looks like their heads are sticking out of their chests. Some develop huge humps in their upper backs. Do you need x-rays and scientific evidence to tell you that this spine has changed for the worse? That it's rigid and works like an old rusty hinge on a gate left out in the rain for 50 years? Is it a coincidence that so many other parts of their bodies fail miserably as well? That their hips and knees and feet have grossly distorted through the years? How about their bowels and digestion? Sexual function? How can any of these things possibly work right when the nerve supply to them has been compromised for decades?" He paused a moment and added, "X-rays are a valuable tool, but I don't see a need to x-ray every baby and child. With some experience, your hands and eyes tell you very clearly what's going on in someone's spine."

He took a deep breath and sighed loudly. "Do you think it's just luck or genes that allows one 80-year-old to joyfully play tennis while another sits in a wheelchair drooling?

I interrupted again, "Isn't a lot of these old timers' problem simply arthritis?"

He looked at me sternly. "Arthritis is the *result* of a subluxated spine. Leave the tension and the reduced range of motion in the body and the natural result is arthritis. Better yet, let the stresses and tensions of life *accumulate* in the person. Arthritis is an *effect* of a failing system. Arthritis is the body's attempt to adapt to the aberrant mechanics, tensions and imbalances in the system. You can treat the arthritis until you're blue in the face, but unless you get the tension – *the subluxation* – out of the system, the arthritis will be there. And it *will* get worse. Drugs may ease the symptoms, but leave the spine subluxated, and the end result is the little old lady or little old man who can barely walk or get out of a chair."

He paused a moment, then continued. "It amazes me that people and doctors alike never ask why one hip or one knee is grossly arthritic and the other is fine. If it were genetics, it would be both, right? If it were just old age, it would be both. Aren't both hips the same age? If it were due to an old injury, why didn't it heal? When the pelvis and/or spine are subluxated, it causes hips, knees, ankles and feet to adapt and change to the increased tension and decreased motion. That adaptation expresses itself as abnormal mechanics which is the underlying cause of most arthritis.

"So, do you know what brings these poor individuals to the point of severe pain and immobility? Ignorance and neglect. Ignorance of vertebral subluxation and its devastating effects on the human body, and neglect of the care of their spines. That's why I continue to go from town to town speaking and teaching chiropractic to anyone who'll listen." He shook his head slowly. "You see little old ladies go to the beauty parlor once a week to make their hair look pretty, but their spines? Completely neglected. And men? They take better care of their cars than they do of their bodies. A hunk of steel that they'll probably have for six or seven years, and they understand the importance of *its* maintenance. Meanwhile, their spines decay and they wonder why they can't do the things they used to."

He noticed my blank expression and smiled. "I'm not unsympathetic to them, Adam. I've made it my life's work to teach people about chiropractic so they can live more healthfully and don't end up crippled and dependent on multiple medicines to get by. And keep in mind; chiropractic care of the spine and nervous system involve so much more than just physical ailments. Subluxations affect how we think, how we feel, how we sleep, how much energy we possess throughout the day, and how well our organs and glands produce all the proper chemicals for every activity in the body. One little uncorrected subluxation caused from a mildly traumatic birth or a little bump on the head at age two, and the health and vitality of that person goes downhill from that point on."

"This brings us back to the original point of why I use these old timers with the grossly distorted spines as my example. When people doubt the concept or existence of subluxation, I ask them if they notice the changes in the old-timer's spine. Of course they do. OK, I ask, just when and how did it start? At age 70? 50? 30? 12? I'll tell you. In the vast majority, it started very young. Fortunately, the body adapts amazingly well when we're youthful and relatively strong and flexible. So when did it start? After the car accident or slip on the ice? During the troubled childhood? After the traumatic divorce or bankruptcy? Usually, it's an accumulation of *multiple* stresses and traumas endured throughout life.

"You don't think these things affect the spine and nervous system? Think again. Can't you just see the way some people hold their necks, shoulders and backs? Can't you just see the tension in their faces, or in the way they walk, breathe and move? Subluxations are very real and very common, even in young children. And they're *so* easy to correct when addressed in infants and children."

He frowned. "This is the saddest thing to me. Here's little Suzie, two years old, and she's got a little subluxation of her atlas. That's the first vertebra, the bone right under the base of the skull. It's shifted just slightly to the right. She and her parents don't notice it, and of course, no pediatrician in the world would notice it. It would take a minute or two, maybe a few adjustments to correct. But leave it alone, and wait until she's 25, and now it's not so easy. Her body has made all kinds of adaptive changes in response to that one little subluxation. Leave it uncorrected until she's 50 or 60, and her spine is basically a mess. Tight, rigid, arthritic, painful. She's anxious all the time. You've heard the expressions – *tightly wound, high-strung, a bundle of nerves.* And don't forget about all the other problems that this little subluxation has created during her life – neurological, immunological, organic and glandular. But now she's 55, and she can't turn her head to see if a car's coming when she pulls out of her driveway, so she is convinced by a friend to see a chiropractor. A few adjustments and she doesn't feel any better. *This isn't helping me,* she thinks.

"Do you see what I'm getting at, Adam? I'm not saying poor Suzie can't be helped. Of course she can. Every person is better off with a more highly functioning spine and nervous system. Always. Without exception. It's late, but it's never *too* late. It's just that it would likely take years to get her spine functioning properly again. Many years. That's not an easy thing for most chiropractors to tell someone, and that's partly why so many choose to treat her symptomatically instead. And so in a few weeks or months, her neck feels better, it turns a little easier, and off she goes. Or it *doesn't* feel better, or maybe even feels worse after an adjustment or two and she never goes back to another chiropractor again. She winds up going back for more drugs, more injections and more surgeries."

He scowled. "This reminds me of a personal story. I was traveling through New Mexico about 10 years ago, and stopped to get adjusted by a friendly young chiropractor. He spoke of correcting subluxations and wellness care, so I thought I had made a wise choice in asking him for an adjustment. Well, he practically took my head off. It was the most violent adjustment I had ever received in more than 50 years. When I questioned him about it afterwards, he said that his technique was designed to *permanently* correct the subluxation in one or two visits. I thought, *you better hope one, because I can't imagine anyone coming back to you for a second visit.* We talked for a while, but I couldn't convince him that his adjustment was too rough. I couldn't get him to explain his *permanent* correction or his concept of subluxation either. He saw it as something stuck in time and space and his extremely forceful adjustment *fixed* it.

"This is a problem I've noticed through the years; too many chiropractors are too rough. They're hurting people, and then they wonder why the people don't come back. I think perhaps because B.J. Palmer was a forceful adjuster, they assume it's the way to be. But if we chiropractors scare away half the people we see, what's the point?"

I blurted out, "I thought you said that chiropractors don't hurt people."

"I don't mean hurt in the sense of injured. I mean just using too much force and being too rough. Some people are very sensitive and chiropractors need to be aware of individual tolerance. The skilled chiropractor has hands that can feel the tone within each patient and match his adjusting skills to the individual, rather than using the same degree of force on everyone. There are many gentle techniques in chiropractic and I feel that every chiropractor should learn and master both gentle *and* forceful techniques."

We pulled into Uncle Earl's driveway. I helped him unload the car, and he told me I could sleep in the guest bedroom upstairs if I liked.

"I guess I'll spend the night at the Sprague's since my stuff is there, but I'd like to stay with you tomorrow night if that's okay. Then I'm going to head back east on Sunday."

"Sounds fine, Adam. What are your plans for tomorrow? Are you up for some early morning kayaking?"

He knew that I was an avid outdoorsman like himself, so he wasn't surprised when I quickly said, "I'd love to. What time should I be here?"

"Six o'clock." He gave me a big hug and we said goodnight.

During the drive back to the Sprague's, I thought about my knee injuries and surgeries, my asthma and my headaches and tried to see the connection between them and my spine, pelvis and nervous system. *Could it really be as simple as Uncle Earl said?* I studied anatomy and physiology and know how complex the human body is. And the brain? No one fully understands its vastness. But the biggest thing I still couldn't understand is why my father, and medical science in general, doesn't acknowledge, or at the very least, research the basic premise of chiropractic.

At the bed and breakfast, I packed up my clothes and guitar, loaded up my pickup, and went to the front desk to pay my bill, assuming no one would be around at five-thirty in the morning. "Hi, I'm Colleen", said the strikingly beautiful woman behind the desk. "You must be Adam Hale." She looked about 40 and had long, dark brown hair and sparkling, brilliant green eyes. I detected an Irish accent as well.

"And you must be Irish," I blurted out unconsciously. I wasn't shy, but I realized it sounded odd. I tried to soften my bluntness, so I added, "Your eyes look just like one of my dear friends who's 100 percent Irish. "I'm sorry. Yes, I'm Adam Hale. Pleased to meet you."

"As a matter of fact, I *am* from Ireland, but I've lived in Colorado for the past 15 years. Pleased to meet you too, Adam."

She handed me my bill and it read *No Charge*. I thought it must be a mistake, but before I could speak, she said that Sam and Edna were happy to have me stay, and since I was Earl's nephew, they wouldn't charge me. I wanted to thank them, but she said they'd already gone to bed.

"Do you get adjusted, too?" I asked, anticipating her lovely brogue.

"That's why I'm in Southold Springs," she said. "I live about two hours south of here, but I've been staying at the inn for the past few months."

"You're a guest at the inn?"

"Well, I work here at the desk and clean and do laundry for the Spragues, and they let me stay here so I can get adjusted from the Hales." She saw my puzzled look and continued. "Sam and Edna have done this for years. They allow people to stay at the inn for weeks or months so people like me can receive chiropractic care for an extended length of time. If you have a minute, I'll tell you my story and how your family of chiropractors saved my life.

"About 12 years ago, I was exhausted all the time. I had no energy at all. My doctor diagnosed me with CFS – Chronic Fatigue Syndrome – and put me on two medicines. Well, I gradually got worse, so he sent me to a number of specialists. Some said it was CFIDS – Chronic Fatigue Immune Deficiency Syndrome – and others labeled it fibromyalgia. Test after test and procedure after procedure and not one doctor was certain about what was wrong with me."

"How many doctors did you go to?" I interjected.

"Thirty-three different doctors, mostly specialists. I even spent a week in the Mayo Clinic. Every part of my body ached all the time, and I was so weak that I couldn't even walk to the end of the driveway to get the mail. I became very depressed, which caused some of the doctors to think I was a head case, and so they sent me to psychiatrists as well. At one point, just a couple of years ago, I was on 11 different medicines. I wanted to die. I spent all my time in bed, crying and feeling very sorry for myself. It took all my strength just to get up to go to the bathroom."

She paused and smiled at me. "One day, my sister had a friend visiting from Southold Springs, and said that I must come here to see Dr. Earl. I told them both that I couldn't face one more doctor, test or procedure, but her friend convinced me that this was different, and that it sounded like my nervous system could use some real help. They made all the arrangements, and the three of us drove up to Southold Springs about 10 weeks ago."

"You don't look sick to me. In fact, you look really healthy."

She laughed. "I am now, but you should have seen me then. The first time I went to visit Dr. Earl, I was in a wheelchair. After only four or five adjustments, I could feel some life returning to my body, and after a month, I took myself off all of my medicines and started to walk again. Slowly at first, and just around the house, but little by little, I regained my strength, and now I can walk up and down these steep hills of this beautiful property. I walked for two miles yesterday, and even jogged a little bit. My head is clear, I have energy, and I'm smiling again for the first time in years. You have no idea how great it feels to be able to perform simple tasks like doing a load of laundry or making a bed again. And although I feel so very blessed for my new life, I'm pissed as hell at all those doctors for never sending me to a chiropractor." She blushed a little and added, "Please pardon my French."

We both laughed and she added seriously, "I suffered for more than 10 years and now, in less than three months, I'm alive and well thanks to chiropractic. I've got my life back. So that's my story, Adam. I am eternally grateful for your wonderful family of chiropractors."

I didn't know quite what to say, so I just smiled.

We said goodnight, and I went right to bed, looking forward to kayaking in the morning.

*The law of the absolute
must be obeyed or one must reap pain and anguish.
The law is: never criticize; never find fault;
never abuse; never blame anyone,
either to his face or behind his back;
never hurt anyone's feelings – man or animal.
Never permit harsh or unkind words
to escape ones' lips.
Instead, speak words of love, of trust
and of kindness.*

Paul Twitchell

7

At six a.m. I arrived at Uncle Earl's doorstep. He greeted me at the front door and asked me to park my pickup around back. We got in his Jeep and headed north to Turquoise Lake. After some small talk, we stopped at a cozy little diner for breakfast.

As soon as we walked in, I heard *Mornin' doc*, and *Hey Earl, goin' fishin'?* He introduced me to Jerry, the owner and chef, and Joyce, a middle-aged waitress with long, braided, grayish-brown hair. She looked weathered, as if she'd had a hard life. As we walked towards the counter, Joyce grabbed my arm firmly and said loudly to me, "Do you know what your uncle did for me 20 years ago? I had kidney failure and was on dialysis for eight years, three days a week. They said I would have to be on dialysis for the rest of my life. Well, my lower back was so tight and painful, so I went to Dr. Earl thinking he might help me. That night, after my very first adjustment, I peed, not like a racehorse, mind ya, but I peed for the first time in eight years." Uncle Earl and I sat down and she gave us menus while she continued to talk. "I called up my doctor the next day, and you know what he said? He said it was impossible for me to pee 'cause my kidneys didn't work. After a few months of adjustments, I never needed dialysis again." She leaned over and gave Uncle Earl a big kiss on the cheek. "I'm alive and well because of your uncle, Adam."

Uncle Earl smiled humbly and said to Joyce, "Tell Adam what the urologist said to you when you told him that you peed. It's classic." He laughed.

Joyce looked directly at me and said, "You're not gonna believe this, but he said that it was impossible for me to pee, and I better stay away from the chiropractor 'cause he *hypnotized* me into believin' I peed."

She walked away humming the Beatle's song playing on the radio, and I looked at Uncle Earl, thinking of Colleen's story last night and Joyce's this morning. "Do you have some incredible gift, or healing ability or something?" He smiled and said, "No, Adam. I simply remove interference in the central nervous system. The *credible* healing ability is in each and every one of us. It's called *being alive*. Remember that innate intelligence I spoke about?"

We ordered omelets, toast, juice and coffee. Uncle Earl sipped his coffee and said. "Please don't misunderstand, Adam. There are lots of reasons for kidney failure, such as genetics, toxins, drugs, alcohol, parasites. Joyce is an example of subluxation-caused kidney failure, meaning that apparently the reason her kidneys stopped working was due to interference in the nerve supply to them. It's actually quite simple. She injured her back in her early teens, got subluxated at the level of T11-T12, that's the 11th and 12th thoracic vertebrae, and gradually, the nerves from that area in her spine – *which lead directly to the kidneys* – were damaged, eventually causing the kidneys to stop functioning."

He asked Jerry while he cooked our breakfast, "Hey Jer, if you put those four pieces of bread into the toaster, pushed them down, and went back to check them a minute or two later and the toaster was cold, what's the first thing you'd check?" Jerry let out a big laugh and said, "You can't fool me, Doc; I'd check the plug. You teaching Adam some chiropractic?" Uncle Earl laughed too, and replied, "Yeah, thanks Jerry."

Uncle Earl turned back to me and looked serious. "Do you know how many doctors Joyce went to when her kidneys began to fail? More than a dozen. They tested her left and right, up and down, x-rays, CTs, MRIs, IVPs, blood, urine, you name it. All over the country. All these brilliant men and women, dedicated specialists, and not one thought of *checking the plug* to her kidneys." He sipped his juice. "Every person who's ever studied the human body knows that the major nerve supply to the kidneys comes from the level of the 12th dorsal vertebra. So why don't they check it?" His voice rose. "Why don't they even *consider* the nerve supply to a malfunctioning organ or gland?" He took a deep breath and exhaled with a little groan.

I asked, "If chiropractors can cure kidney disease, why don't all the people on dialysis go get adjusted?"

He smiled at me and spoke very slowly. "Adam, chiropractors don't *cure* anything. They correct subluxations to restore balance and harmony to a neurologically impaired body, and the better-functioning body heals itself. There is no curing. I suggest people get that word out of their vocabulary and mind. Little or nothing gets cured, except perhaps a ham." He smiled at his own joke. "I've seen the commercials; this *cures* athlete's foot. No it doesn't. It may temporarily alleviate the symptoms, but the athlete's foot usually returns in a few weeks or months. Healing is much bigger than curing. Healing is something done *by* you. Curing is something done *to* you. Healing is an internal, natural process that living organisms undergo every moment of their lives. Curing is the illusory *fixing* of a condition from something outside the individual."

He sipped his juice. "Should every person with kidney failure get adjusted? Of course they should. To improve their nervous systems, their bodies and their lives. But there's no guarantee that it will have any impact on their kidney disease. Like I said before, there are many reasons for kidney failure.

"And don't get me wrong. I'm not criticizing or blaming the doctors for not checking the spine or nerve supply. It's not in their training, and sadly, not even in their thinking. I try to enlighten and inform them just as I try to educate everyone else. Some are open and receptive, others not at all. Many medical doctors refer their patients to chiropractors. Many do not."

Joyce served our food and filled our coffee cups. Uncle Earl thanked her, and then said to me. "Remind me to tell you of the Winsor autopsies later. For now, enjoy your breakfast."

While we ate he told me of the different kinds of wildlife we might see while kayaking. I enjoyed Uncle Earl's company. His joy and love of life certainly were obvious, and he laughed a lot, too. His mannerisms reminded me a lot of my father's, but Uncle Earl seemed much more relaxed and at peace with life. And his passion for chiropractic seemed boundless.

He paid for breakfast so I left the tip. We thanked Jerry and Joyce and headed for the lake.

Before I could remind him, he said, "In 1921, there was a medical doctor from Pennsylvania named Henry Winsor who performed autopsies on 75 human and 22 cat cadavers to determine if there was any correlation between the cause of death and the region of the spine related to the diseased organ or gland. I'm not sure if his motivation was to prove or disprove chiropractic, but he was extremely curious about all the claims that chiropractors were making in those days. He decided to do some real research on the spine and its relationship to disease, and the University of Pennsylvania gave him permission to carry out his experiments. Back then, some very bold chiropractors claimed that by adjusting specific vertebrae they could *cure* specific diseases. Keep in mind that in 1921, chiropractic philosophy was still evolving."

I interrupted, "Don't some chiropractors today make similar claims?"

"Yes, unfortunately they do. I believe that the wise chiropractor should stick to the simple truth that we set the central nervous system free, which allows or helps the body to heal itself.

"So if a person died of heart disease, Dr. Winsor would examine the area of the spine from where the nerves go directly to the heart. Lungs, pancreas, kidney, stomach, colon. Whatever the person or animal died from. Guess what he discovered? That in more than 90 percent of cases, there were specific areas of spinal and nerve damage at the corresponding spinal region. All nine cases of stomach disease showed spinal misalignments in the fifth through ninth thoracic vertebrae. All 26 cases of lung disease, all 13 cases of liver disease, all 17 cases of kidney disease, and all 20 cases of heart disease. As for the prostate, uterus and spleen, all showed corresponding damage at the spinal levels involved as well. He may have undertaken this project to disprove the chiropractic principle, but he ended up scientifically validating chiropractic instead. Common sense doesn't require proof, though. Doesn't it make perfect sense that if the major nerve supply to the stomach comes from the level of the sixth and seventh thoracic, and that area of the spine is injured or subluxated, that there will be some sort of neurological deficit to the stomach?"

"But 1921? I doubt it was a peer-reviewed experiment."

"Good point, Adam. True, but this is why I appeal to the use of logic and common sense. If you had a sick child, would you wait for scientific validation? There's no real science behind the removal of hundreds of thousands of sets of tonsils in the last 70 years, but surgeons did it, and *still* do it anyway. It's not science at all. It's simply, *let's cut out this child's tonsils because we've exhausted antibiotic therapy and don't know what else to do.*

"About 20 years ago, I was at a dinner party with some friends. One couple, visiting from out of town, mentioned how they had been trying unsuccessfully to conceive for more than four years. They'd visited half a dozen specialists, been through every test and procedure imaginable, spent thousands of dollars, but no pregnancy yet. I mentioned to the husband, who happened to be a physician's assistant, if he'd checked his wife's third lumbar vertebra, and he snickered condescendingly at me. Of course, the friends that knew me knew how serious I was. I asked Allison if she'd had any spinal problems, and she said 'none whatsoever', although she did say that she had hurt her lower back once in gymnastics when she was a teenager. She was a marathon runner and appeared in great shape. I asked if I might run my hand down her spine gently and she said okay. I pressed into each lumbar vertebra, L1-5. All felt fine but the third lumbar. It was rotated to the left, and when I touched it, she nearly jumped off her chair. 'Ow! Why does that hurt so much?' she asked. I didn't have to answer. A few of my friends blurted out 'subluxation', and we all had a good laugh. I explained a little chiropractic to her, pointing out the fact that the primary nerve supply to the ovaries and uterus comes from the level of the third lumbar vertebra. Since they were only visiting for a few days, I suggested she come in the office. I adjusted her third lumbar three times and two months later we got an extremely happy and grateful phone call informing us that she was pregnant."

I was puzzled. "I still don't understand why medicine doesn't embrace the chiropractic principle if it's as great as you say it is."

Uncle Earl sighed and gathered his thoughts. "Forget embracing. It's very difficult for medicine to even *acknowledge* the basic principles of chiropractic. You see Adam, as I mentioned last night, if they were to acknowledge that even *one* person's health improved, or *one* organ or gland improved in function due to a chiropractic adjustment, then logically, they would have to acknowledge the fact that every person, under every circumstance, is better off with a clearer nerve supply, free from vertebral subluxation.

"This isn't rocket science, Adam. We're not dealing with complex mathematical formulas here. There are 24 vertebrae in the spine and from in between those vertebrae exit the spinal nerves, which go *directly* to and from the organs, glands, muscles and every other part of the body. They are direct and obvious pathways. It's like a car hitting a utility pole in front of your house and you can't understand why your lights and TV don't work. Hey, the power's out because the electricity's been cut off!

"But can you picture the decree from the American Medical Association?" He smirked and continued. "OK doctors, no matter what part of the body is malfunctioning or diseased, we want you to check the person's spine for subluxation, and if you don't know how, send the person to a chiropractor to make sure his nervous system is working properly first. *Then* proceed with proper medical protocol." He laughed quietly at his own sarcasm and added, "Sadly, that would actually be much better for the health of the population, but if you're going to wait for medicine to prove, accept or understand what we do, you'll probably die waiting."

He could see by my face that I still couldn't fully understand why more people didn't know about this. "It's really a philosophical difference, Adam. Medicine, in the last few hundred years, is blood chemistry-based and steeped in outside-in, mechanistic thinking. By that, I mean that not only do they look *outside* the body for remedies or cures, but they look at diseases as things or entities that attack the body from the outside as well. Look at cancer. It's perceived as a *thing* that some unfortunate victim *gets*. Listen to the language used referring to cancer. *It* went from her breast to her liver. *It's* in her bones now. She's got *it* in her brain. Cancer is not really a thing or entity. It's a *process* by which the body's cells reproduce out of control or erratically. It's a *manifestation*, an *effect*, of weakness, confusion or improper function in the body.

"A study in the New England Journal of Medicine conducted by the University of Copenhagen found that adopted individuals had the cancer risk of their adoptive parents, and *not* their biological parents. Genetic factors account for less than 15 percent of the cancer risk. So what are the major factors?"

I thought for a moment, but before I could answer, he spoke. "First, a weakened immune system. Subluxations weaken the immune system, and are likely the most overlooked factor in all of medicine."

I grinned and said, "So if I get adjusted regularly, I won't get cancer?"

"I would never say that. But I *do* know that your nervous and immune systems will work more efficiently, and that is probably the greatest deterrent to cancer you can have."

"Why is that?"

"Cancer is uncontrolled cellular growth and reproduction, so common sense tells me that it's wise to keep the system of the body that maintains control over cellular growth and reproduction – *the nervous system* – working optimally. And that means regular chiropractic care. Better nerve supply, greater control. So I would say that you are *less likely* to have cancer, but there are no certainties or guarantees in life, other than death and taxes."

"You mentioned the word *mechanistic* again. What do you mean by that?"

"Partly that mechanists see the sum of the parts equaling the whole. By dissecting and examining every part of the body, mechanists think they can understand the entire body. We vitalists believe that the whole – meaning the person, the being – is *greater* that the sum of the parts. Consciousness, thoughts and feelings cannot be seen, touched or measured in a laboratory, but they are a big part of what make us human and unique. And they are *huge* factors in determining our ability to heal and recover, as well as our overall levels of health and happiness."

He pulled off the road to stop at a gas station with a mini-mart inside. While inside paying for gas and snacks, a tall, rugged-looking man in line in front of us talked to the cashier about his various ailments. His skin looked like the leather of his tool belt, so I assumed he was a construction worker of some kind. I noticed that he was buying two different medicines, along with two packs of cigarettes and a cup of coffee. "My arthritis is sure killing me these days," he said to the disinterested cashier. "And this time of year always makes my allergies worse, so I have to take this stuff every day." He pointed to one of the medicines. "Is this the strongest stuff you got for allergies?" Although I heard his words, I didn't give them too much attention.

In the car a few minutes later, Uncle Earl asked me about the rugged man's language and what I thought about it. "I don't know. He looked like a pretty tough middle-aged guy to me."

Uncle Earl glared at me. "His *language*, Adam. His choice of words." I wasn't sure what he was talking about, and my silence and blank expression showed it.

"The words a person uses reflect his state of consciousness or awareness. Words are a reflection of how we think, and how we think affects every aspect of our lives, including health, finances and relationships. Our choice of words speaks volumes about who we are. For example, his use of the word *my* in describing the allergies and arthritis. What does the word *my* infer?"

After a brief moment, I answered firmly, "Ownership, possession."

He smiled and said, "Exactly. When we put the word *my* in front of any condition or disease, we *own* that condition or disease. And ownership of any condition makes it a heck of a lot harder to rid oneself of that condition. Ridding oneself of a condition is called healing by the way, and it happens from the inside out. When you were a kid and broke your arm, it healed, right? The condition – *the fracture in the bone* – no longer exists. The problem is that the vast majority of people mistakenly equate healing with curing. They think that taking a medicine to ease the symptoms or effects of a condition is removing the condition. It isn't. It's simply offering temporary relief *from* the condition. Also, keep in mind that the doctor may set the bone and place the arm in a cast, but it's the intelligence within the body that does the actual healing."

Uncle Earl merged back onto the highway. "Let's get back to those few little sentences uttered by the man at the gas station. And please don't misunderstand; I'm not judging the guy. I'm just using him as an example regarding the importance of words. The reason you didn't recognize anything unique in his language is because his choice of words is extremely common. *My* arthritis. *My* allergies. *My* colitis. *My* migraines. You hear it every day. But remember, your words and thoughts are a reflection of who you are and how your life works. And the idea is to have your life work as well as possible, which brings us to his next word, *killing*. Do you think it's wise to say something like, *my arthritis is killing me today*? It's not. It's a very destructive choice of words. It hurts your body and mind every time you say it. *My back is killing me. My head is killing me.* People say it every day, along with things like; *I have a bad back*, or *bad knee or shoulder*. Do you think it's wise to call a body part *bad*?"

I asked quickly, "But aren't these just harmless expressions? I mean, it doesn't *really* hurt you to say those things, does it?"

He pursed his lips and glared at me again, reminding me of my father when he was serious about teaching me something. "Yes, Adam, it *does* hurt. Science has actually demonstrated that our thoughts and words affect our body. Your thoughts and words can raise and lower your blood pressure, and they can even raise or lower your white blood cell count, which means they affect your immune system. This is real, Adam. It's not new-age mumbo-jumbo, and the sooner you understand this, the more responsible for your own health and well-being you become. Happiness and positive words are extremely powerful tools to help strengthen your immune system, as well as your entire body and mind.

"Words and language are expressions of thoughts, and thoughts are things. Although not 100 percent accurate, lie detector machines pick up the slightest changes in our thoughts, which produce energy, and in turn create change in matter. So think good thoughts and your body will be better. Simple. Just because we can't see thoughts doesn't mean they're not real. We can't see electricity, but we know it's there and we can see its effects. Thoughts have effects too, and those effects manifest and can be seen in the quality of our lives."

He smiled at me, giving me a moment to absorb his words, and then continued. "*My arthritis is killing me* also places the responsibility *outside* oneself, reinforcing a victim mentality. It's as if you were an innocent bystander and arthritis jumped out from behind a bush and latched onto you, as though you had nothing to do with it. In truth, you created it. Something you have done or have not done allowed the joints of your body to become inflamed and degenerated. Sadly, most people don't understand that arthritis, like most diseases and conditions, is a *process* and not a *thing.* To label a disease and consider it an entity empowers the disease and disempowers the individual."

After a minute of silence, he asked, "Adam, are you aware of the concept that what we think and talk about expands?"

"I read Napoleon Hill's book, *Think and Grow Rich,*" I said.

"Wonderful. Many people, Deepak Chopra, Norman Vincent Peale, Wayne Dyer and others have spoken and written about this idea for centuries. Emerson wrote, *a man is what he thinks about all day long.* I am a strong believer in this concept. I believe we attract to our lives whatever is in our current dominant thoughts. So when people continually think and talk about their pains, conditions, diseases, medicines, surgeries and doctor visits, do you think this makes them healthier?"

"I guess not."

He frowned at my vague response and said, "It actually makes people sicker. These people rarely heal from anything. Instead, they get more of what they think and talk about. In fact, some people identify so strongly with their disease or condition that no matter what they do, it's nearly impossible for it to leave their lives. They either learn to live with it or try to control or manage it with drugs. And instead of looking within for answers or considering that they might have the innate ability to heal, they wait for medicine to find a cure. And sadly, they usually die waiting.

"I don't mean to offend with these words, but what do you think might happen when an entire island with a population of a few million people continually talk about conquering or curing breast cancer? You would think that those people would have a relatively high rate of breast cancer, and guess what? They do. Keep talking about it, keep raising awareness and money for it, and you'll likely have *more* of it. It's kind of a strange catch 22. People think that they're helping conquer the disease by increasing awareness, but there's a good possibility that they're actually creating *more* of the disease. This isn't an easy thing to tell people – that quite possibly, every time you donate or contribute to curing cancer, heart disease, Parkinson's, Alzheimer's or something else, you're actually *feeding* that disease. You're adding to it, helping it grow by giving it attention and energy in the form of money."

"That sounds a little weird, Uncle Earl, and I think you might hurt or even infuriate some people with this kind of talk."

"Then let's put it this way – if you want *more* of something in your life, think and talk about it continually. This is why I strongly recommend that people get out of the habit of continually talking about their pains and illnesses. If you really want more health in your life, talk about health, vitality, energy and life. Use words like great, wonderful, dynamic, vibrant, and radiant referring to your state of health. Positive attitudes, thoughts and words go a long way in the healing process. And if these words aren't part of your language, it's pretty likely that they're not part of your life, either."

I blurted out, "Are you suggesting people not support medical research and the curing of diseases?"

"I'm just saying that I believe in the principles of attraction and attention, and that I don't see any diseases being cured. Billions of dollars and tens of thousands of researchers, and nothing really gets cured. Sure, treatments are better and many lives are made more comfortable, but curing diseases? Nonsense. It's like dangling the carrot in front of the donkey's nose, except they're taking huge sums of money and leading people on with marketing terms like *advances, breakthroughs* and *groundbreaking research.* With modern medicine, today's breakthrough is often tomorrow's lawsuit. People, especially in the United States, are sicker than ever. My heart goes out to the individuals and families suffering, but when I see a celebrity on TV say something like, *we're getting very close to a cure for Parkinson's or Alzheimer's or Multiple Sclerosis or Muscular Dystrophy or cancer,* I cringe. It would be laughable if it weren't so sad."

I became adamant. "How can you say nothing gets cured? What about smallpox, polio, diphtheria and tetanus?"

"Okay. You're referring to vaccines now. We'll get into them a little later, but for now I'm referring to the false hope and faith that are placed in modern medicine and the language we've been cultur-ally conditioned to use."

"Isn't hope good for people?" I asked.

"Yes, I believe it is. But lying to the public with statements like, *we're very close to finding a cure,* is wrong." He paused in thought a moment, then added, "One of the worst and most insidious things the pharmaceutical marketing machine does to people is keep their attention focused *outside* themselves. The cure, miracle, treatment, therapy and restoration of health all come from without. *It,* the answer to our problem, condition or disease, exists *outside* our bod-ies, and it comes from them and them alone in the form of a drug or treatment. This takes the person's attention away from the greatest doctor and healer in the world, the innate intelligence, the life force within.

"And don't think it's just the medical community that thinks from the outside inward. Many in the holistic, new-age and natural healing models are of the same consciousness, but instead of drugs, they use plants, herbs, vitamins, algae, seaweed, bee pollen, crystals and dozens of other things. But the thinking is still outside-in. This herb will fix your allergies. This seaweed will cure your asthma. This remedy will cure your arthritis. The same consciousness, but with different tools.

"And I don't believe God or nature hid the secrets to health deep in the Amazon Rain Forest or in algae found two miles below the ocean's surface. It's not to say that these substances don't help certain people sometimes. I'm sure they do, and I take various herbs and supplements occasionally, but I don't place more power in *them* then I do in my own innate power."

He paused a moment, then asked, "What do you think the constant bombardment of drug commercials does to the conscious-ness of a nation? The daily and persistent mentioning of arthritis, indigestion, asthma, allergies, depression, constipation, diarrhea, cancer, heart disease, and so on keeps the attention of a nation on sickness. And this is exactly what the pharmaceutical industry wants. They want you in their drug stores regularly buying their products, so they need to continually remind you of your conditions and diseases. Where your attention goes, energy flows. So we wind up with a country that thinks and talks about all these diseases and conditions on a daily basis, and it makes us sicker and sicker. It's one of the most subtle, yet destructive brainwashing techniques used in modern times. As far as I know, only the United States and New Zealand allow drug advertising on television, and it will be a great day in this country when it's no longer allowed.

"Do you know why we removed alcohol and cigarettes from television ads? Because they were bad influences on our children. Well, guess what? Drug advertising is a bad influence. To teach young people that the answers to their problems, aches, pains and conditions all lie in pharmaceuticals is bad. It leads to irresponsibility, weakness, sick-thinking and an excessive dependency on drugs."

It felt odd asking, but I said, "You're not one of those conspiracy theorists that believes modern medicine wants to keep people sick so they can keep making money, are you?"

He laughed and answered, "No Adam; I'm not. I believe most of the people doing research, as well as most people in medicine and all the healing arts have the best interest of their fellow man at heart. But I also believe that in the past 50 years the pharmaceutical companies have become huge, profit-motivated corporations. Fifty years ago, most pharmacies were small mom-and-pop businesses. Prescriptions were rare and usually short-term. Nowadays, there are huge pharmacies on just about every corner all over the country, and they're filled with people taking multiple, lifetime prescriptions.

"Individuals and businesses pay for advertising for one purpose, to sell their products. And I believe that if their products – drugs – were really as good as they claim, they wouldn't need to advertise them daily, or at all, for that matter."

"But Uncle Earl, even *you* have to admit medicine does a lot of good for people."

"Of course I know some medicines and surgeries save and prolong lives. I'd never argue that. I simply state that the healthier your body and mind are, the fewer drugs and surgeries you need. Hey, unless it's an emergency, try changing your lifestyle or try chiropractic for six months to a year. You can always take drugs or have surgery down the road. Sadly, due to the magnitude of the pharmaceutical companies' marketing campaign, we take more drugs and have more surgeries and end up with less health and happiness. Drugs and surgery should be the last resorts, not the first."

I challenged, "What if somebody has really high blood pressure, like 220 over 120? You're saying they shouldn't take medicine?"

"That's certainly high blood pressure. I'd say that person is in or near a state of emergency, and that's where medicine is at its finest. But I'd also say that just because his blood pressure is that high on that particular day doesn't mean he needs blood pressure medicine for the rest of his life." He paused a moment and added sternly, "And I *never* tell people *not* to take medicine.

"A few years back, I adjusted a 75-year-old patient who had been on hypertension medicine for 30 years. After four months of chiropractic care, her blood pressure dropped so low that her physician took her off the medicine. She's maintained normal, healthy blood pressure, *without medicine*, for the past three years."

"High blood pressure? Really?" I asked surprised.

He glared at me. "Yes, hypertension. Hyper means too much, and tension means tone. There's too much tension in the blood vessels. And after all I've been teaching you, you're surprised that chiropractic adjustments reduce excessive tone? Hypertension is often a direct result of vertebral subluxation causing increased tension in the central nervous system, which controls the dilation and constriction – the *tone* – of blood vessels."

I asked, "Do you see chiropractic emergencies in your office?"

"To a principled chiropractor like me, every subluxation is an emergency. The sooner it's addressed and corrected, the better the person's life is. A baby with an asymptomatic atlas subluxation – that's the first cervical vertebra – is no less critical than a guy in agony who's brought in on a stretcher. I don't see the man in severe pain as any more of any emergency than the subluxated child with no pain. Why? Because we are more concerned with subluxation and function rather than pain and symptoms.

"Adam, what words do we use to describe modern medicine's attitude towards disease?" Before I could answer, he said, "Ever hear of the *war* on heart disease or the *battle* or *fight* against cancer? We try to *conquer* flu, the common cold and other conditions. You get the idea. For thousands of years, we've been battling diseases, trying to eliminate them from our lives to make the world a better and healthier place." He added sarcastically, "How are we doing with that?"

I grinned sheepishly. "I guess not too well, at least in the U.S."

"The World Health Organization claims that 80 percent of all diseases are created by our attempts to conquer disease. What happens when you declare war on something? You get more of it. In 1972, President Nixon declared war on crime. Guess what happened during the following decade? Crime rates went up! How are we doing with that war on drugs? Or trying to eliminate rats, cockroaches and mosquitoes? Psychologist Carl Jung said, *what you resist, persists*. It's the law of attraction in reverse. When you resist something, it's still in your mind, which keeps it in your life. Fighting something does not get rid of it, but keeps it around instead, and will often attract or create even *more* of it."

"So are you saying we shouldn't fight diseases?"

"Well, medicine has been hell-bent on conquering diseases for a thousand years, so I doubt they're going to stop now, especially with their current ability to create extremely powerful drugs. Look at the many species of bacteria that are almost totally resistant to antibiotic therapy today. They adapt faster than we can create the drugs to kill them. Medicine thinks the answers all lie in pharmaceuticals and in the control, containment or destruction of all the bad germs and they're very likely to continue on that path, in spite of their obvious failure. But individually and as a society, I think rather than fighting disease, it's wiser just to become healthier.

"Yes, I realize that sounds silly and simplistic, but we get more obese, lazy, and unhealthy and drug-dependent by the day. What's not understood in the world today is that one of the best ways to improve health and happiness is to improve the function of the body and mind with chiropractic care. Chiropractic is not a substitute for a healthy diet, fresh air, water and movement, but it *is* the huge missing link in health care today.

"Louis Pasteur, considered by many to be the father of the germ theory of disease, had an adversary named Antoine Beauchamp. Pasteur stated that germs caused disease, while Beauchamp said it was the state and condition – *the terrain* – of the host that determined disease. Shortly before he died in 1895, it is reported that Pasteur acknowledged and agreed that it was more the host than the germ, and yet the germ theory still permeates and dominates our society today. It's easier and less responsible to blame sickness and disease on something *outside* us. We've been doing it for centuries.

"Also, realize that it's always easy to blame things we cannot see. For centuries, the cause of sickness and death was demons and evil spirits, and the doctor had to exorcise them from the patient, using all kinds of bizarre treatments. When the first bacteria were seen under a microscope, a new cause was discovered. Then came the electron microscope and viruses became the culprits. Sadly, even to this day, the condition of the host, *the person's constitution*, is rarely considered by medicine.

"In 1950, conjoined – Siamese – twins were born in the Soviet Union. Masha and Dasha were joined at the pelvis and had four arms and three legs. Each girl controlled one leg, and the third leg dangled behind them, and by age five, they learned to walk. They could not be separated because they shared too many organs and systems. They shared the same circulation, which meant that any virus or bacteria that got into their bloodstream was in *both* of them. Yet one girl frequently got sick and the other didn't. Sadly, the twins were used in medical experiments because the doctors couldn't understand how one could remain healthy while the other was sick. Colds, flus, measles and other diseases affected one girl and not the other. One eventually got cancer, which caused both girls to die at age 19. By that time, the medical researchers concluded that the only possible reason one got sick while the other didn't was the fact that they had separate central nervous systems – separate brains and spinal cords. These doctors discovered that the state of the central nervous system was the determining factor regarding health and sickness. Imagine that."

Uncle Earl drove while I admired the mountains and rapidly moving, white-capped river parallel to the right side of the road. The sunrise in the mountains cast an orange and golden glow to the east. I thought about his words and my own fear of germs as we turned onto a narrow and rough dirt road, lined thickly with evergreens on both sides. Then my uncle said, "Exactly one mile up this road is the cabin. The road's a bit rough on the Jeep, but it's worth it. Wait till you see this place."

Within a few minutes, the trees opened onto a clearing, at the center of which stood a beautiful, modern log cabin and a spectacular view of a large purple-blue lake, bordered by rugged mountains. It looked like a post card. As we pulled up to the cabin, we startled a flock of geese. As the geese flew over the lake, I saw three large elk bound into the thick woods, effortlessly clearing a hedgerow of four-foot bushes.

The Jeep stopped and I immediately jumped out. My mind reeled with words to describe the magnificent sight, but all that came out was "Wow!" The lake was as smooth as a mirror. The air was brisk, but so clear. Uncle Earl stretched outside the Jeep and said to me, "It's a beautiful day and we're lucky to be alive. Take a few deep breaths of that mountain air and tell me life's not grand." I took a deep breath and smiled.

The cabin was equally beautiful inside. "You can tell your aunt did the decorating," he said. It had a warm country charm, with a sofa and loveseat that matched the deep red plaid blinds and curtains. The adjacent kitchen was modern and spotlessly clean. The view out the picture window was spectacular. With each bit of increasing daylight, the lake gradually got bluer and brighter. All I could think was, *this is exactly where I'd like to live someday.*

You are as old as your spine.

Paul Bragg

8

There were six kayaks in the backyard. We dragged two down to the water's edge, grabbed our paddles and life vests, and loaded up our coolers and binoculars. Uncle Earl taught my brother Mike and me to kayak when we were very young, and it's remained one of my favorite pastimes. I was accustomed to kayaking the salt-water creeks and bays of eastern Long Island, so I greatly anticipated the stillness, flora and fauna of a fresh water lake. There was nothing I'd rather do on the Fourth of July weekend.

We paddled out slowly, and Uncle Earl spoke almost immediately. "If you don't mind Adam, this morning I'd like to teach you about what I consider to be much of the heart and soul of chiropractic, and the great missing link in modern medicine and health care – the relationship between structure and function in the human body.

"A few weeks ago, I saw a 70-year-old woman I had adjusted a few times about 30 years ago. Back then, she had some mild low back and neck pain, and after those few adjustments, she felt much better. Although I tried to teach her the importance of regular chiropractic care so her spine and pelvis would have a chance to improve, heal and function properly for the rest of her life, she didn't think she needed any more care because her pain was gone.

"She told me that in the past five years, she had both hips and one knee replaced, *and* lumbar disc surgery. She is bent over and walks painfully with a walker. There is no doubt in my mind that these surgeries and her disability could have been avoided had she taken care of her spine 30 years ago. Instead she, like many others, thought *my back feels better; why do I need more adjustments?* And so she never got adjusted again. In her mind, she put chiropractic in the medical Band-Aid model. So when her back pain returned in a few months after I adjusted her, she went back to her medical doctor and got more drugs for pain, inflammation and spasm. And the rest, as they say, is history. *Her* history. And sadly, millions of others like her as well. Why? Because nobody thinks it's going to happen to them, *especially* people who practice yoga, run, swim, or do some other kind of regular exercise. But my 40-plus years of experience in adjusting people has taught me that it happens to most spines that don't receive regular chiropractic care throughout their lives. It's gradual, subtle and so common.

"If the mechanics of the pelvis and spine are aligned, balanced and working properly, the discs and joints stay healthy. The hips and knees will be healthier as well because they will move in their normal ranges of motion. If there is a subluxation present, meaning misalignment along with increased tension and restricted or aberrant joint mobility *anywhere* in the spine, moving parts will wear and tear prematurely. The moving parts in the human body are called joints, where one bone meets – *articulates* – with another. There are about 300 joints in the human body, and 101 of these joints are in the spine and pelvis, and they are easily and frequently injured throughout our lives.

"Now don't get me wrong. Should I ever need a hip or knee replacement, I would be extremely grateful for the great minds that designed it, and the great skill of the surgeons and staff that did the actual surgery. These people, like many others in medicine, do amazing, life-saving and life-improving things every day.

"But that said, medicine doesn't seem to understand or acknowledge the fact that if proper mechanics are restored to an injured joint, that joint can heal. Instead, they usually see the joint as arthritic, treat it superficially with drugs, and watch it slowly degenerate until surgery or joint replacement is necessary. When they see a patient with a hip or knee problem, they rarely look at the spinal and pelvic structures and their relationship to the hips and knees.

"Here's a statement I hear all too often from people, and sadly, often in their 50s and 60s: *the orthopedist said my hip, or knee, is worn down to bone on bone.* Doesn't it make sense to address these mechanical derangements *before* they've reached bone on bone? Isn't it easy to see that the problem started years or decades earlier?

"Mechanical, joint, problems, don't happen randomly. They happen due to very specific and sometimes obvious causes. Trauma is an obvious cause, but that leads to the question of *why didn't it heal?* Vertebral and sacroiliac subluxations are the most likely reason for spinal, pelvic, hip and knee joint problems, as well as the primary reason a joint doesn't heal fully after an injury. Changes in the position, tension or mobility of the spine, pelvis and spinal cord alter mechanics. By its very definition, a subluxation is a change in the mechanics."

"What do you mean by *why didn't it heal*?" I asked.

"I can't tell you how many times I've heard people say something like, *my knee is bad because I injured it playing high school football. Or gymnastics. Or an old war injury or car accident.* And my question to them is; *why didn't it heal?* It's a simple question. Many people have broken bones in childhood and the condition, *the fracture*, doesn't exist any more. Why? Because the bone *healed.* The innate intelligence of the body repaired the broken bone and within weeks or months, it's as good as new. Do you think the wisdom of the body can heal broken bones, organs, glands and tissues, but forgot how to heal the joints of the back, hips and knees?"

I mumbled a weak "No", but knew not to interrupt him when he was on a roll. "Okay Adam, so *why* didn't the injured joint heal? *Why* is the hip or knee still a problem 20 or 30 years later? *Why* did it get worse with time instead of better? The reason a joint doesn't heal back to healthy is usually due to faulty mechanics. It's physiologically impossible for the joint to heal when it's continually under duress. By the way, it's often the same spinal or pelvic subluxation that created the initial weakness in that joint, allowing it to be more easily injured.

"Let's take the example of a 12-year-old boy who keeps re-injuring his knee on the soccer field. He goes through physical therapy, cortisone injections and two arthroscopic surgeries, and no one among the pediatricians, orthopedists, PAs and PTs has made the connection between the spinal/pelvic distortion and the chronic knee problem. And so his knee gets examined, x-rayed, treated, drained, injected and surgically cleaned up, and no one has looked at, *or even considered*, the spinal and pelvic postural and biomechanical dynamics that very likely created the weakened and dysfunctional knee in the first place. And so the kid goes through life with not only chronic subluxations, but also a chronic knee problem."

We smiled at each other, knowing he was speaking about me. "He thinks he's unlucky or just has a bad or weak knee. Or he simply blames the original injury. Actually, he's stuck in a mechanistic, medical model of thinking that unintentionally encourages or at least allows the mechanics of the body to continue to break down. The joint is labeled arthritic and worsens over time instead of healing, so he continually tries new and different medicines and procedures to ease his pain. He and his doctors never seem to realize that you cannot correct a mechanical problem with a chemical solution. It simply makes no sense. Greasing the misaligned front end of a car does not solve the problem. It must be aligned.

"The knee is a simple flexion joint. Well, *no* joint in the body is really simple. They're all magnificent designs. But by simple I mean that it doesn't have the complex range of motion like a hip, shoulder or spinal joint. Although the knees rotate slightly, basically, knees flex and extend much like a hinge or the knuckles of your fingers. The femurs, thighbones, sit on top of the tibias, shinbones, and along with strong collateral and cruciate ligaments and medial and lateral menisci, which act as cushions; there are your knee joints. Each knee is designed to support about half the body's weight. Hence, the menisci, the cushions. Now imagine the knee joint slightly misaligned due to changes – *subluxations* – in the spine and pelvis. Can you see how it would be more prone to injury? Can you see why it would continue to deteriorate no matter what is done to the knee itself?"

I thought of all the medicines and cortisone shots I took over the years. "Don't anti-inflammatory drugs help minimize joint damage by reducing inflammation?"

"Maybe temporarily. But know that inflammation is part of the body's natural healing process. And although it's true that excessive inflammation can sometimes cause damage to tissues, taking an anti-inflammatory medicine goes against the innate intelligence of the body. I believe the healthy body knows exactly how much inflammation to produce according to the injury. The innate intelligence of the body also knows exactly how much cortisone to produce to help that knee heal. Also, if these drugs help arthritic and degenerating joints, why don't the millions of people on these drugs get better instead of gradually getting worse, usually leading to surgery or joint replacement? Remember that we're always talking about *healing*, and not simply pain or symptom removal. If the objective is to heal, or at the very least minimize or repair joint damage, the best thing you can do is make sure the joint is moving in its normal, healthy range of motion. *Aligned and free.*"

"Why doesn't medicine understand this?"

"The medical model is familiar, like one's religion. When you grow up thinking a certain way, it's difficult to imagine anything else. Medicine has been treating mechanical problems with chemicals for 100 years with no success, but they still do daily research to find that wonderful, miraculous drug that will one day cure arthritis and joint pain once and for all.

"I'm being facetious because it's absolutely ridiculous to think it's possible for a drug to correct a joint problem? A joint is a hinge. It's *completely* mechanical in nature. The root Arthro *means* joint. *Arthr*itis means joint inflammation." He laughed lightly. "I read recently that some medical experts believe that they will have the cure for arthritis within 10 years. How can you possibly cure something you don't understand?

"Recent studies have shown that most arthroscopic knee surgeries, as well as most spinal surgeries, are ineffective, especially over the long term. They cost us billions, but do little to nothing to improve lives. Why? Because they treat the *effects* of degeneration and not causes.

"I've heard it said by some orthopedists that a meniscus can't heal on its own. I've heard some say the same about the intervertebral discs in the spine as well. You know what I say to that, don't you? Ridiculous. Nonsense. I believe the innate intelligence of the body is capable of healing *any* part of the body. Of course if the doctor's experience is to never see anyone's discs or menisci heal, it follows that he's going to think it's not possible. And if the alignment, the mechanics of the joint, is left unchanged by treating it only with drugs, therapies and exercises, it *will* continue to degenerate and not heal. Exercise in these cases actually accelerates the degenerative process for obvious reasons.

"It's absolutely ludicrous to think that the body, created miraculously from those two tiny half cells, can heal broken bones, injured, torn, or cut skin or muscles, damaged organs and glands, but somehow, it just can't heal discs or knees. How unreasonable does that sound, Adam?"

I stared at him, thought about my knee, and realized it made sense. "But didn't you say that chiropractic is vitalistic and not mechanistic?"

He smiled at that. "Yes. But we work *with* the mechanics of the body to free the nervous system and allow the innate intelligence of the body to better express itself. We are vitalistic because we see the life expression and healing ability in every cell and tissue and seek to allow free and unrestricted communication among all parts of the body. We don't just see a kid with a knee problem and look at the knee *only*."

We both watched in awe as a Golden Eagle flew silently overhead. He continued. "When we're born, our spines are in a C-shaped curve from neck to pelvis. In the first few years of life, two secondary curves develop. These are the forward, or lordotic, curves of the neck and low back, which add a lot of strength and flexibility to our spines. In order for these curves to develop properly, the pelvis, which consists of the sacrum, coccyx and two innominate bones, must be structurally and functionally sound."

I interrupted, "Innominate bones?"

"Some call the innominates *hipbones*, but the hip is actually the ball and socket joint created by the head of the femur, the ball, and the acetabulum, the socket, of the innominate bone." He placed his paddle across his lap and patted both hands on his sides by his back pockets and said, "These are your two innominate bones, the big bones that make up the majority of the pelvis.

"The development of normal, healthy spinal curves is essential to proper energy utilization, proper postural adaptation and proper spinal neurobiomechanical efficiency. The pelvis is the support and base for the entire spine, and when it is subluxated, even slightly, spinal development suffers, and health is diminished.

"The primary function of the pelvic musculature is not movement, but rather pelvic stabilization and the maintenance of proper, balanced distribution of the weight load. The pelvis is all about maintaining a balance between the upward forces generated through the feet and legs and the weight of the body from above. And from our very first steps as toddlers, these forces literally grind our sacroiliac joints into shape. By the time we're three or four and running around like normal kids, the biomechanics of our spines and pelvises are pretty well developed.

"A Nobel laureate by the name of Roger Sperry, M.D., said that 90 percent of our brain's energy is used for posture alone. The remaining 10 percent is for thinking, metabolizing and healing. So if you're spine and pelvis are even slightly altered in those first two or three years of life, your brain and body will use more energy for posture and the rest of your health and life will suffer. This is why chiropractic care is so crucial for infants and children. When the spinal or sacroiliac joints are subluxated in early childhood, the spine develops improperly, and instead of a healthy, fully-functional spine, we end up with one full of imbalances, adaptations and compensations."

I interrupted and asked, "How do infants get subluxated sacroiliac joints?"

"Great question. Primarily trauma. As a child learns to walk, he or she falls at least 50 times a day. Babies fall from high chairs and changing tables. Emotional stress and trauma causes changes in the tension and positioning of spinal curves, as well as spinal and pelvic function. One study of 650 young children showed subluxations and aberrant mechanics in 96 percent of their pelvises. And what do these changes in spinal and pelvic dynamics lead to? A lifetime of weakness and diminished health and function. More drugs, more surgery, less life and less joy.

"Adam, do you think arthritis develops in a healthy joint? No, it doesn't. Look at my knuckles. They all move in their full range of motion with relative ease. And so do my hips, knees, shoulders and everything else. Joints are designed to function well for a lifetime of 100 years if they're taken care of properly."

"Is it true that cracking your knuckles causes arthritis or big knuckles?"

"No. Moving joints is good for them. Joints are designed to move. I've cracked my knuckles 20 times a day for the last 60 years and they're absolutely fine. They're not enlarged or arthritic at all, and they all work as well as they did when I was 10 years old. Isn't that the idea, Adam? To keep every joint in the body working as well as it possibly can? It certainly makes life better when you can move with more ease. This is why I believe taking a drug to ease joint pain, and that means backs, necks, shoulders, wrists, hands, hips, knees and feet is counterproductive to healing. It's truly the *wrong* thing to do. Sadly, the millions of people taking these drugs have no idea that they are actually contributing to the degenerative process in their bodies. By taking the medicine, they give themselves the *illusion* that things are better while nothing is done to actually improve mechanics and function."

"What exactly is the noise when you crack your knuckles?"

"To the best of my knowledge, the cracking is simply due to the expansion of the joint capsule. It causes a little carbon dioxide to be squeezed out of the synovial – or joint – fluid. It's kind of like opening up a can of soda. Some of the carbon dioxide quickly leaves the fluid, causing a little pop. It takes about 10 minutes for the synovial fluid to absorb carbon dioxide back into it, and then you can crack the joint again. It's not the cracking that's important; it's the overall effect on the joint. Is its range of motion better? Does it move easier and smoother? Have the muscles relaxed around it? As a joint improves in its range of motion, the soft tissues around it, meaning the muscles, tendons and ligaments, can now all work with greater ease. I think people made up those lies about it causing arthritis or big knuckles simply because they didn't want their kids cracking their knuckles all the time. And instilling fear is a great way to get people to stop doing something. As long as it's not done violently, cracking your knuckles is fine.

"And it's the same with adjusting the spine, which sometimes causes the cracking or popping sound. I've heard and read that some orthopedists and physical therapists, usually in a lame attempt to attack or criticize chiropractic, have stated that too much *cracking* of a joint can cause joint damage or hypermobility. My experience with thousands of people and millions of spinal adjustments, as well as with my own body, tells me that they're wrong. I've seen hyper-mobility in the spine, but it's usually due to an adjacent subluxated or fixated vertebra. Most commonly, the first and second cervical vertebrae subluxate and cause the fourth, fifth and sixth cervical vertebrae to compensate and become hypermobile. That's precisely why they frequently demonstrate the obvious disc problems and facet joint arthritis. And it's the same with a fixated or subluxated sacroiliac joint; it causes the fourth and fifth lumbar vertebrae to take up the slack and that's why those joints and discs commonly deteriorate."

I interrupted. "I once heard one of my dad's friends, an ortho-pedic surgeon, say that chiropractic can injure discs of the spine. Is that true?"

"No. Intervertebral discs are so strong it would be difficult to injure one if you tried. Most disc problems are due to years and decades of gradual wear and tear from improper mechanics

– subluxation. Like water dripping on a rock over time, it will eventually wear the rock down. Chiropractic adjustments actually *improve* the integrity of the discs because they improve the integrity of the joints and the spine as a whole."

I felt odd asking this question, but did so anyway. "This same doctor once said that chiropractic has a placebo effect and only works when people believe in it. Is there any truth to that?"

Uncle Earl chuckled and then seriously said, "Nonsense. Ignorant nonsense. I've adjusted dogs, cats, birds, a rabbit, an iguana, and hundreds of babies, and I've seen profound and wonderful changes occur after delivering those adjustments. When a three-month-old baby with severe colic gets adjusted and his colic is gone for good the very next day, it didn't happen because the baby believed it would. It happened because the principle of chiropractic is scientifically sound and logical. When a subluxation is reduced or corrected, the body works better.

"But speaking of placebos, do you know that your grandfather and many other medical doctors of his time used placebos in their practices? Why? Because they worked. They gave sugar pills to patients, and those patients got well because they believed they were taking medicine. Do you know why doctors *don't* use placebos any longer? Because they work, and because they don't want to lose credibility and control by prescribing sugar pills. Along those same lines, studies have shown that people believe that when a medicine is very expensive, it must be better medicine."

Like most people, I never gave too much thought to the mechanics of the spine and pelvis, but I needed to ask, "Is there proof in medical journals of these causes of arthritis and spinal degeneration?"

"Yes Adam, loads of it. I can show you books and dozens of published papers from all the major medical journals that refer to the mechanical breakdown of joints and discs, but I'd rather appeal to your logic and common sense. Keep in mind that most of what passes for science in these journals is not truly scientific. And just because a research paper is peer-reviewed and published, doesn't prove that it's scientifically sound either. Do you know of Archimedes, who lived about 2,000 years ago?"

"Didn't he have something to do with physics?"

"Yes. Archimedes is the father of mathematical physics, and he discovered the principle of displacement that states that the upward buoyant force exerted on a body immersed in a fluid is equal to the weight of the fluid the body displaces. Archimedes' principle is considered a *law* of physics, and is an important and underlying concept in the field of fluid mechanics. There isn't a scientist alive today that doubts this principle. And yet it can't always be proved. Why is that?" He reached into his pocket, pulled out a coin, and tossed it into the lake. "Archimedes principle states that I just made the water in the lake rise the exact volume of that quarter. But can you prove it? No, because it's impossible to measure. There are miles of shoreline and lots of nooks and crannies, and simply no way to measure that tiny volume of water I just displaced.

"And so it is with chiropractic. There isn't a machine or the technology available today to measure the quantity and quality of the billions of nerve impulses connecting the brain to all the cells, tissues, organs and glands of the body. And yet science has proven that interference in the nervous system certainly disrupts its function. Simple, common sense tells us that it's not a good thing to interfere with the transmission of nerve impulses in the human body."

He took a deep breath and sipped some juice. "Let's get back to other effects of faulty mechanics. Do you think calluses, corns, bunions and heel spurs develop for no reason? Are the people who get these things unlucky or genetically inferior?" Without waiting for an answer, he continued. "Again, spinal and pelvic subluxations cause the body to adapt and compensate. These foot problems, as well as many others, *are* the body's adaptation to changes in weight bearing, balance and tone. To *subluxation*."

I interrupted. "Doesn't exercise or yoga prevent a lot of these problems?"

"Exercise and yoga are wonderful, but they don't prevent or correct subluxations. And they are certainly no substitute for chiropractic care. Remember, our spinal and pelvic curves, postures and tones develop very early in life, and I've never met a one or two-year-old who exercises. As a matter of fact, exercising on a subluxated, imbalanced structure will actually *increase* the rate of joint degeneration. I've seen marathon runners with gross pelvic distortions, and I cringe when I think of the damage they are doing to their bodies. It's like driving the car with a misaligned front end faster and farther to try to *work it out*. It's only creating more wear and tear. I implore runners and all athletes to get their spines checked and adjusted regularly. Even if you're only slightly off, you're not doing your lumbar spine, sacroiliac joints, and hips and knees any great favors. Sure, your heart and legs are strong, but see the bigger picture. The spinal and pelvic biomechanics are so important, and yet overlooked by so many so-called experts. And keep in mind, we're still only talking about mechanics. Chiropractic's greatest impact is on the central nervous system. But for now, let's continue with mechanics.

"Many people think because they exercise, do yoga, or eat healthful foods, that they don't need chiropractic care. But subluxations are often present in the most apparently healthy people. I've adjusted professional athletes and yoga masters as strong and flexible as the contortionists in the circus, and have found subluxations present in their spines.

"X-rays don't lie. If you were to randomly x-ray the spines of a thousand people between the ages of 40 and 50, you'd likely find significant disc and facet joint degeneration in the majority. Any radiologist will tell you that joint and disc degeneration are *so* common in the mid-cervical spine and the lower lumbar spine. They see it every day. And remember, it's often painless for months and years, so the diminished mobility, weakened, subluxated joints and gradually degenerating discs are usually ignored, considered normal, or attributed to aging. And of course, when they *do* become symptomatic, they are treated wrongly with drugs and other temporary, superficial means.

"People rarely picture themselves 10 or 20 years older than they are at the present moment. For example, a 20-year-old with a mild backache doesn't think about spinal biomechanics, vertebral subluxation, and what her spine will be like at 40. She thinks her back is just stiff because she played tennis or gardened yesterday, has her period, or slept in an awkward position. And she certainly doesn't think that her little back pain might cause her right knee to need arthroscopic surgery at 40 and complete joint replacement at 55. But that's how it happens. Sure, people have serious accidents that require surgery and joint replacement, but the vast majority of joint surgeries are due to the *gradual* wear and tear from subluxations that occurred in childhood. Most back, neck, hip and knee surgeries are entirely preventable."

"I read an article recently in which surgeons proudly claimed that within the next 10 to 15 years they will be performing four to five times the number of hip and knee joint replacement surgeries they're doing now. They made it sound wonderful. Well it isn't wonderful. What would be really wonderful would be these doctors and patients becoming aware of and properly addressing the spinal and pelvic mechanics *before* the joints wore down to the point of needing replacement. There's your greater miracle; *avoiding* joint replacement surgery." He paused to admire a flock of geese overhead, then asked, "What do the majority of people do when they experience a little pain or stiffness in their neck or back?"

I knowingly responded, "They take drugs to alleviate the symptoms."

"Exactly. When a person takes a pill, whether a painkiller, muscle relaxant or anti-inflammatory medicine to ease the symptoms of back or neck pains, they are missing the point. The point of healing and health care is to *be* better, not just *feel* better. The body creates the pain and discomfort to tell us something is wrong or needs to be addressed. I believe that taking a medicine to remove symptoms is usually the worst thing one can do. Why? Because you are ignoring the body's warning system, and only addressing the symptoms rather than the actual problem. Ignoring or masking a mild symptom in any part of the body is the best way to create bigger problems down the road. I boldly proclaim that the vast majority of people who have endured spinal injections, back surgery, hip and knee joint replacements have grossly ignored their pelvic and spinal problems throughout their lives.

"Many years ago, Tom and Ray Magliozzi, known as the Tappet brothers, or Click and Clack, told a story on their radio show about a young woman driving to college. Her dashboard *check engine* light, sometimes called an *idiot* light, was on for the duration of the trip. The light bothered her, but instead of investigating and addressing the problem, she covered the light with black electrical tape. It turned out she needed oil, but ignored it and ended up with a seized engine instead. It's not wise to ignore or mask symptoms.

"An important point to understand is direction. In which direction is your body going? By that, I mean that once people are subluxated, their bodies and minds are going downhill, regardless of the presence, absence or severity of symptoms. Taking drugs only masks problems, without actually doing anything to make the body *function* better. So when you take one or more of these drugs, pain-killers, anti-inflammatory or muscle relaxants, *you* are still going downhill. And if you are like most adults, you've been subluxated for years or decades, and x-rays will usually confirm this. You will clearly see the effects of long-term subluxation; disc and joint degeneration, regeneration and narrowing, inflammation and arthritis. Remember, it's all a gradual process. And so is healing. The body can heal these damaged tissues, but it usually takes many months or years. This is why six to eight weeks with a chiropractor or therapist of any kind isn't remotely enough to make genuine progress to most adult spines. You can't undo in a month or two the damage nature has done over decades. Regular chiropractic care is essential to get these spines, pelvises and central nervous systems moving in a positive, healing direction and working optimally again.

"Nothing in nature stands still. You are either moving forward or backward. A peach reaches full ripeness and then begins to rot. Many of us start rotting from early childhood and as long as we remain subluxated, we will never get to experience vibrant health.

"Keep in mind that many spines will never fully heal due to the severity and length of time they've been subluxated. These people can still improve, or move in a positive direction, but they may never completely recover. Also, a small percentage of people have congenital defects in their spines that can cause instability and other problems. But the idea is that no matter what you've been through in life, no matter what you've been diagnosed with, and no matter what anyone has told you regarding your prognosis, chiropractic can still help you."

I asked, "Aren't a lot of back problems muscular in nature?"

"No. Changes in muscle tone are part of the body's adaptive response. It's extremely rare for muscles to be the primary problem.

But doctors and therapists often tell people that they just have a muscular problem, and that most backaches and other musculoskeletal problems take care of themselves on their own. If that's so, then why is the number of people with arthritis increasing? Why are more spinal surgeries and hip and knee joint replacements done each year? Why do millions of people have chronic joint and disc problems and spinal and lateral stenosis, or narrowing, in their cervical and lumbar spines? I'll tell you why – because as a society, we haven't learned that chiropractic care is vital to every spine. We've learned that modern dentistry is important for care of the teeth, but the spine? Nope. People erroneously think that masking symptoms is the way to go because that's what they've been taught by modern medicine and all that pharmaceutical advertising.

"And it's true, a lot of people have back or neck pain for a few days or weeks and those aches and pains often disappear without doing anything at all. But the body adapts and compensates, and the body and mind get accustomed to pain. Most of these people find that their bouts of pain and stiffness generally become more frequent and more severe as they age. Very few actually improve and heal without chiropractic care. How can they when they are left subluxated?

"Just look online, or in any newspaper or magazine around the world. There are always dozens of new treatments, injections and surgical procedures for back and neck pain. It's always *after the fact* treatment. The person is *finally* so debilitated or has endured so much pain that he or she will succumb to almost anything just to feel better. So there's a huge market out there for these poor, uninformed folks." He paused, then added, "How sad, but how unnecessary for the most part. Chiropractic care throughout childhood and life would likely prevent 90 percent of these procedures and surgeries. Instead, people will spend billions every year hoping for that magical cure in a pill, injection or scalpel."

I asked, "So what's the initial cause of most back problems?"

"Subluxation. Spinal and pelvic joint injuries that have never fully recovered or healed. Here's a simple and common example – an infant falls on her butt and mildly injures one of her sacroiliac joints. The joint is a little stuck and only moves about 75 percent of its normal range of motion. No one notices that her right foot turns out a little bit, or that her right hip is a little stiffer than the left. Perhaps a slight scoliosis is detected when she is 12, but that's been developing for years as a result of the small original injury. She has no pain, but the slightly diminished motion of the sacroiliac joint leads to gradual degenerative changes in the hips, knees and lumbar spine. Of course during this process there are always changes in muscle tone and function as well as neurological deficits that may manifest as organ, gland, or immune system weaknesses. The process continues for decades, often with little or no symptoms, and at age 35 she is told she has some arthritis and disc degeneration in her back. Do you get the picture? Of course she never thinks it's going to happen to her, especially if she eats well and is fit and trim. But subluxations happen to athletes *and* couch potatoes alike."

He paused for a while to admire a small fish that jumped out of the water between our kayaks. "If you are doing any repetitive exercise like running, walking, stair-stepping or anything similar, you darn well better make sure you're on a frame that's balanced and free of subluxation. If not, eventually the body will tend to sprain, strain and tear more easily. And if you're a professional athlete and *really* push the body hard while subluxated, you'll wear out even quicker, and probably endure more severe injuries.

"Every year, there are thousands of people with serious spinal injuries which result in paralysis. This is not an easy thing to say, but it's my belief that some of these poor folks are subluxated and therefore more prone to serious injury. Whether it's a football player hitting an opponent straight on with his helmet, or someone in a car accident, if your neck is subluxated, and its natural forward curve is straightened or reversed, it's predisposed to more serious injury. And straightened and reversed cervical curves are *extremely* common, even in children."

I thought about a friend from college who was injured in a motorcycle accident and is now quadriplegic and on a respirator. "That sounds strange, Uncle Earl. You're saying that these injuries could have been avoided with chiropractic care?"

"Some of them, Adam. Sometimes it's simply the great force that causes the fracture, but sometimes it's the poor positioning of the vertebrae – the *subluxations* – that contribute to the fracture." He took a deep breath and continued. "Let's say I've got two sticks in my hand. Both are three feet long and a half-inch thick, but one is green and supple, fresh from the tree, while the other is old, stiff and brittle. If I jam them both into the ground, what happens?"

I visualized the two sticks and said, "The brittle one will likely break, and the green one will bend."

"Exactly. If you're in an accident of any kind, you want your spine to bend. Chiropractic care enables your spine to stay green, supple and more flexible so you are less likely to be injured in the accident. Make sense?"

I nodded in agreement. "Yeah, it does."

"Pardon the crude example, but it's like a drunk in a car accident. He often walks away from the accident because he's loose.

"Some people appear to do everything right. They eat well. They maintain their ideal weight. They don't smoke or drink. They exercise regularly, get lots of fresh air and water, and they think healthy thoughts. And yet they wonder why they *still* have a chronic back, knee, hip, stomach or other body part that is always bothersome. The great reason why is that they have likely neglected the spine. They have missed the two most important pieces of the puzzle, the spine and central nervous system. Increase the wear and tear, the degenerative process to the spine, and you are looking at a long downhill path, regardless of everything else you do. If you're working or exercising with a spinal and pelvic structure that is not sound, *you are deteriorating.*"

"But aren't running and walking good for you?" I asked.

"Yes, provided the joints of the spine, pelvis and lower extremities are sound. But if they are even slightly imbalanced or restricted due to subluxation present *anywhere* in the spine, then walking and running will aggravate the involved joints. Perhaps one knee will adapt and its medial meniscus will take the majority of the burden, causing its premature breakdown. Perhaps both feet and ankles will compensate by pronating or forming large bunions. When there are imbalances and restricted ranges of motion involved due to subluxation, the body adapts as well as it can. But in spite of these adaptations, the degenerative process continues."

I thought of the many tourists I'd recently seen in the national parks. "Isn't obesity a big part of back problems?"

"Certainly it's a factor, but let's use the front end of the vehicle example again. If the front end of a pick up truck is out of alignment, do you think putting 400 pounds of cement in the back is going to help? Of course it isn't. The excess weight is not the problem, but if you are subluxated, obesity will increase the rate of wear and tear for obvious reasons."

"Uncle Earl, if the body is as intelligent as you say, why does it allow the arthritic degeneration to take place?"

Uncle Earl gathered his thoughts and spoke. "Let's say I'm slicing vegetables and I cut my hand accidentally. We've all experienced that. The body forms a scab where I cut myself. What would happen if I picked off the scab? The body would have to go through the entire healing process again, right? It would have to send fibrinogen and other clotting factors to the cut and form another scab. The pulling off of the scab *disrupts, irritates and perpetuates* the healing process. Theoretically, I could continue to pick at the scab and keep that cut open for months or years. Well, that's exactly why some backs and knees and other parts of the body don't heal. The innate intelligence of the body *tries* to heal the injured part, but can't catch up with the ongoing duress. That's why I say that arthritis is the *result* of a problem and not the problem itself. It's usually the body's attempt to heal the very best it can under its current conditions. And it's my strong belief that the living body is *always* doing everything in its power to make and keep us healthy and strong. That's why we chiropractors address *interferences* to our natural state of health and function.

"Chiropractic helps people in two ways – first, mechanically. When the joints of your spine and pelvis are balanced and move in their normal, healthy and full ranges of motion, your life is better. You move with more ease. Your muscles are more relaxed. You have fewer aches and pains. You need less medicine. You need less surgery. Second, and most importantly, your central nervous system works better. As important as the mechanics of the spine are, chiropractic's greater benefit to mankind is its positive impact on the central nervous system. Common sense – *and science* – tells us that when your central nervous system works better, every aspect of life is better. Your thinking is clearer, your brain chemistry is better, your emotions are more balanced, and every organ, gland and system in your body functions better."

He pointed out the Golden Eagle's mate on a branch 30 yards away. I looked through my binoculars and gasped in awe at its huge size and brilliant golden-brown color.

He continued. "The word *disease* came from dis-ease, meaning a lack of ease. A healthy body is one that works with *ease*. Don't we all want more ease in our lives? Don't we want to breathe with ease, digest with ease, eliminate with ease, climb a flight of stairs with ease, and get out of a bed or chair with ease? Especially as we get older. Everything we do in life is better with ease, and it all centers around a healthy spine and nervous system. This is what chiropractic has to offer to a very sick and suffering humanity – ease. Medical doctors may be the masters of *dis*ease, but chiropractors are the masters of ease."

We paddled slowly in silence for a while. Uncle Earl pointed out turtles sunning on the banks, fish under our boats and various birds overhead and feeding along the shoreline. Even amidst all the beauty, I looked down at the surgical scars on my left knee and thought about its relationship to my spine and pelvis again. "Uncle Earl, had I been adjusted as a young child, could I have avoided all my treatments and surgery?"

He smiled warmly and said, "I don't know, Adam. Probably, but I never saw your MRIs, so I don't know the extent of your injuries. Most likely your knee problem was due to, at least in part, your atlas subluxation we adjusted when you were 10 years old, and your pelvic distortion."

"I have a pelvic distortion? How do you know that?"

He laughed heartily and said, "Adam, I've been observing and adjusting spines and pelvises for 40 years. A person's tone, breath, posture and movement speak volumes about their spine and health. I can tell a lot about what's going on in someone's spine and pelvis in the first 10 seconds I see them."

"Really? How?"

"Well, the left side of your pelvis is slightly posterior, or backwards, and slightly internally rotated. This causes your left foot to flare out about 10 degrees, which by the way, probably caused, or at least contributed to, your chronic knee problem. Your left shoulder is higher than your right, and your head tilts a bit to the right, telling me that your atlas – the first cervical vertebra – is probably subluxated to the left."

"But I thought you fixed that when I was 10?"

He scowled, reminding me of my father again. "Ah, there's that *fix* word. I *adjusted* you once and you were fortunate to have your asthma disappear, but that doesn't mean your spine was instantly fixed, as you say. Even at 10 years old, it often takes weeks or months to fully correct a subluxation that's been present for years. I suggest you get the words *fix* and *cure* out of your vocabulary, at least regarding the health of the human body. Only pets get fixed, and only hams get cured, and I do neither. I adjust to reduce and correct vertebral subluxations, and trust that the body will *heal*."

"Can everyone learn to read the body like you do?"

"Certainly. Whatever you observe and study becomes easier to understand in time. My entire professional life has been devoted to the relationship between structure and function in the human body, so I can't *not* notice it." We both chuckled at his use of the double negative, but I got the point. He continued. "With knowledge of the way the human body works and a little practice observing it, it's easy to become aware of spinal and pelvic patterns and distortions. Also, I know what healthy looks and feels like. And it's not about perfection, but rather excellence, ease, grace and fluidity, like the spine of a baby or toddler. I've found that when children are adjusted regularly from birth or early childhood, their spines stay amazingly supple and healthy, which allows them to live healthier and happier lives.

"An interesting point that many chiropractors have discovered is that two people may have the exact same subluxations, but they manifest differently. Why? Because there are billions of nerve fibers involved. In your case, the pelvic and cervical subluxations caused bronchial, lung and knee problems. But in another, the same subluxations may show up as stomach and shoulder problems. Yes, pelvic distortions are sometimes the cause of both acute and chronic shoulder problems. The pelvic distortion causes the lumbar spine to adapt by rotating, which causes the thoracic spine to rotate as well, usually in the opposite direction. When the thoracic spine rotates, even slightly, it takes the rib cage along with it, which in turn, alters shoulder mechanics. This is why we chiropractors are less interested in the pain, symptoms and effects of subluxations than in the subluxations themselves. As B.J. Palmer used to say, *we are D.C.'s, doctors of cause.*"

We paddled in silence for about an hour and finally reached Uncle Earl's picturesque log cabin.

*Science is a first-rate piece of furniture
for a man's upper chamber,
if he has common sense on the ground-floor.
But if a man hasn't got plenty of good common sense,
the more science he has, the worse for his patient.*

Oliver Wendell Holmes

9

Back in the cabin, Uncle Earl put on some soft background music and we enjoyed a great lunch together. We talked about the eagles and other wildlife we saw while kayaking. I asked if he could adjust my spine later and he said he'd love to when we got back to the office.

During the drive back to town, I thought about a girl I dated in high school who was recently diagnosed with multiple sclerosis. I asked, "Do chiropractors treat MS?"

"To me, chiropractic is at its very best when it's non-diagnostic and non-therapeutic. By that, I mean that we don't diagnose or treat any specific disease or condition other than vertebral subluxation. So to answer your question; no, chiropractors do not treat MS. We adjust people *with* MS, but we do not treat MS. Why do you ask?"

I told him about my former girlfriend, and that I wondered if seeing a chiropractor might help her.

He asked me, "Do you know what the term *autoimmune disease* means?"

I nodded yes and said, "It's when the body attacks itself, right?"

He smiled and said, "Yes. It's when our own immune system does damage to tissues. What does that sound like to you? What's happening inside that body?"

I grinned sheepishly and looked at him blankly.

He calmly said, "MS is an autoimmune disease in which areas of the central nervous system's myelin sheaths break down and become sclerotic, which means that they harden. You can read volumes on all the theories and research on it in the past 150 years, but medical science still really doesn't understand autoimmunity very well. As with many disease processes, the medical community still doesn't understand causes and what's actually happening."

"And *you* do?" I boldly asked.

He smiled at my boldness, as though he encouraged it. "I'm not claiming to know everything that goes on inside the human body, but I do say that every autoimmune disease is a manifestation of a confused system. If the living body *is* intelligent, why would it attack itself? *Attack* is the word *they* use, by the way. I don't believe the body *attacks* itself, but that's part of medicine's battling and conquering language. I believe something has caused or enabled the body to lose control of its normal, harmonious function, allowing destructive antibodies to be produced when they shouldn't be."

He paused to take a deep breath and asked, "So what system in the body is responsible for controlling and coordinating *every part* of the body?"

"The nervous system." I proudly answered.

"Exactly. And what's the major cause of interference or disruption *to* the nervous system?"

"Subluxation," I answered with less certainty.

"And what type of doctor has the greatest positive impact on the central nervous system by correcting subluxations?"

"Chiropractors."

"Yes, subluxation and chiropractors, Adam. So you've answered your own question. Chiropractic might not just help your former girlfriend, but it may allow her brain and spinal cord to function well for the rest of her life. I've seen many people with MS, and most do very well with chiropractic care. More than a few times, the person has gone back to his or her medical doctor a couple of years later and were told that they were originally misdiagnosed because they no longer had any symptoms or lesions."

I asked, "What about ALS or Parkinson's Disease?"

He scowled at me lightly. "What about them? If I were diagnosed with either, I'd make certain that I wasn't subluxated. The very *first* thing I'd do is get my spine checked. Again, the people with these diseases, as well as the entire medical community, are still looking for that magic drug or formula that's going to save the day and cure these poor souls."

I scowled lightly back. "Hold on, Uncle Earl. What about diseases like polio and smallpox? They're practically gone, thanks to vaccines."

"True, Adam. Perhaps those diseases are nearly gone. But at what cost? Have we traded a dozen childhood and other diseases, some relatively benign, for dozens of other ones? The rates of asthma, allergies, autism, Asperger's, ADHD, Alzheimer's and arthritis have skyrocketed in the past 30 years since vaccination programs were stepped up. And that's just the *a*'s! I realize the link between vaccines and these and other diseases is unproven, but *something's* causing us to become a sicker society. Sure, environmental factors may play a role, but medicine stepped up its mass vaccination program in 1989, and to me it's pretty obvious that injecting *hundreds* of biological and chemical substances into the bloodstreams and tissues of babies is the primary culprit. And I know some people died from the diseases you mentioned, but they die from these other things, too. *And,* some die from vaccines as well. Not to mention the many thousands who suffer every year from reactions to vaccines. Pediatrician Robert Mendelsohn, M.D. asked, *have we traded measles and mumps for cancer and leukemia?* He also referred to mass vaccination as a *time bomb,* meaning that somewhere down the road, the damage from vaccines is going to blow up in our faces."

After a moment of silence he said, "There are more diseases now than ever before. And there are more dedicated scientists and researchers using state of the art technology and spending more money than ever before. But in reality, nothing really gets cured. Why? Well first, the *cause* of most diseases is unknown. Modern medical physiology textbooks are filled with statements like, *it is believed that, it is hypothesized that,* and *current research shows that it may be due to.* The phrase *etiology unknown* is seen throughout the pages of these books, and put simply, it means *we don't know the cause.* Most diseases are still blamed on germs and genetics, and if the cause of a disease is unknown, a virus is often to blame. And second, for the most part, they think only chemically. What chemical formula is going to save us? Or perhaps, what can we do to change the DNA in this person? Or, can we build nano-robots to destroy the bad germs or cancer cells?"

"Are you against nanotechnology, and genetic and stem cell research?"

"I try not to be for or against anything, Adam. Although I'm very passionate about chiropractic, I'm not against medicine. I've often jokingly said that I'm not *anti*-medical, I'm *un*-medical. Genetic and other research will continue, regardless of what I think or say. I'm sure some people will be helped and some will die along the way. It's the way life has always been, and the way medicine has always progressed. I think that sometimes we just want it to be like Doctor McCoy in Star Trek. You know Bones McCoy and Star Trek, don't you, Adam?"

I was a big fan, but surprised that my 65-year-old uncle was. "Sure, Uncle Earl."

"In the movie *Star Trek IV*, the Enterprise goes back in time and lands in modern-day San Francisco. They need to pick up a pair of humpback whales to save the future earth. Well, one of the crew is injured and winds up in a hospital. Bones goes to the hospital to rescue his crewmate, and happens to walk by an elderly woman on a gurney. He asks her what's the matter with her and she says *kidney dialysis*. Bones shakes his head in disgust and mumbles, *Dialysis? My God. What is this, the Dark Ages?* and hands her a pill. Of course, it's always a good idea to accept and swallow a pill from a total stranger." We both laughed. "In less than a minute, we see the woman off the gurney doing a little dance, completely cured of kidney disease."

He took a drink of juice from his cup, sighed deeply and continued with a bit more power in his voice. "Do you see the illusion? Do you really believe that someone can abuse her body for more than 50 years and have damaged, scarred and non-functioning kidneys, but can then take a pill and have perfectly functioning kidneys again in 30 seconds? Please, take me through the process, the mechanism by which taking a pill can restore old, damaged, worn-out cells and instantly create vibrant, healthy ones."

I stared blankly at him.

"Will science occasionally hit on a miracle drug every so often? Sure. If you gave a thousand sick people different parts of a thousand plants, you'd probably come up with a miracle or two. And it's the same with drugs. Sometimes you'll hit on one that has miraculous results. But *individuals* heal; very few diseases are really cured. What makes me angry is the fact that medicine leads people on with the illusion that the cure is close. They want us to think that the near future is filled with wonderful and magical cures for all diseases. But like the Star Trek movie, it's fiction."

I thought of my mom suffering with low back pain and what I'd recently read about chiropractic, so I spoke. "I notice you don't speak of low back pain too much. Isn't that a big area of chiropractic expertise?"

"Low back pain is a symptom, and to a principled chiropractor, symptoms are important to acknowledge, but they have little to do with the location, analysis and correction of vertebral subluxation.

We know that the body produces symptoms for very definite reasons, and we trust that the better functioning body will take care of the symptoms when they are no longer necessary. This is why I believe that seeking symptom relief *alone* for low back pain, or for *any* pain or symptom, is usually stupid."

I laughed. "Stupid?"

"Yes. It's about as stupid as taking the batteries out of a ringing smoke alarm because you don't like the noise. Pain is the noise. Pain is the messenger. Pain is not the problem; it's the body's attempt to communicate with you. The stronger the pain, the louder the alarm, and the more you need to pay attention and step up your awareness. Pain is actually a wonderful gift to help us learn and grow, but we've been erroneously taught to judge all pain as bad and as something that needs to be artificially and quickly removed from the body. People take all kinds of painkillers for years to deaden the messages without ever doing anything to understand what their body is trying to tell them. This leads to the further breakdown of the body and the need for stronger drugs, injections or surgery. The alarm is silenced, and so the house burns down."

I blurted, "But what about people dying from cancer and other diseases? Are you saying they shouldn't take medicine for their severe pains?"

"Of course not, Adam. That's when pain medicine is a blessing. Cancer, trauma, post-surgery, advanced diseases. These people benefit greatly from pain medicine, and I too would be grateful for it if I were in their shoes. I'm talking about the 95 percent of the population who take these drugs for day-to-day aches and pains."

My mom recently went through a series of epidural injections for her low back pain, so I asked, "How do you feel about spinal injections?"

He smiled. "About the same as I do about most symptom care in medicine. After the fact, missing the point, and superficial."

I asked abruptly, "Missing the point?"

"Yes. The point is health, function, vitality. These are the goals of the wise doctor. When the goal or objective is merely the removal of symptoms, the bigger point of health is totally missed. Causes are missed or ignored. Freedom from symptoms is not health. Today, thousands of people with no symptoms at all will die from heart attacks and strokes, or be diagnosed with cancer. They are sick, but because they have no symptoms, we incorrectly think they're healthy.

"I don't want to insult these pain management doctors. I realize that they are performing a service and doing their best to help people in pain, but I see epidurals and other spinal injections as a huge fad in today's medicine. They're another of medicines' experimental procedures that really don't work, especially long term, and cost us a fortune in so-called health care. And you're aware that people are injured by spinal injections every year, aren't you?"

"Yes. When mom went through them, I read up on them online."

He continued. "When people suffer from chronic pain, they'll do just about anything for relief. Drugs, injections, surgery. Now I'm not walking in their moccasins, and I realize that many peoples' spines have reached a point of extreme damage with joint and disc degeneration, stenosis and scar tissue. For these people, the injections may be beneficial, at least for a while. Even temporary relief is a godsend for someone with chronic pain. Sadly, most of these poor folks have relied on medicine throughout their lives to mask the pain of their degenerating spines. And it's usually this long-term masking that has led them to eventually need extreme procedures like spinal injections and surgery.

"Pain management has become a huge field in modern medicine mostly because medicine has failed these people for decades by improperly treating their mechanical problems with chemical solutions. Even the name is strange to me – pain management. Who wants their pain managed? I don't. I want to *heal*. This is why I'm always more concerned with function rather than symptoms. Again, this is why I advocate improving the function of our spines and pelvises *before* they reach this point. For those who have reached this point of chronic pain due to severe degeneration, I realize that my last statement is meaningless, and that injections may be their only option. But understand that the injection of a strong corticosteroid combined with a numbing agent doesn't make any genuine, long-lasting changes to the body.

"Medicine seeks to suppress symptoms, and I believe that the more we suppress in life, the greater the eventual expression we must endure. Put simply, what you *suppress* will eventually *express*. And how does the body express? Excessive mucous production, fever, sweating, vomiting and diarrhea. All are unpleasant, but all are effective ways to rid the body of excess acid, waste and toxins. Prevent the body from expressing, and there's a good chance you're setting yourself up for some serious sickness down the road."

He paused a moment, then asked me, "When you were young, weren't you taught that every time you had one or more of these symptoms you were *sick*?"

I wasn't sure what he meant, and before I could speak he continued.

"When most people experience diarrhea, vomiting, fever or excessive mucous production, they consider themselves *sick*. You missed school because you had a fever. When you returned to school, you told the teacher you were *sick*. But were you really sick? Not necessarily. I think these expressions are signs that the body is working properly, which means healthy. I think they are healthy and necessary expressions of the body and should not be suppressed."

I interrupted, "But what about a child with a fever of 105 degrees? Are you saying you wouldn't address it?"

"Common sense goes a long way, Adam. My children had a few high fevers when they were young, and I'm aware that any of these expressions can lead to serious problems if left unchecked. Prolonged vomiting or diarrhea can lead to dehydration, and very high fevers can cause all kinds of serious problems. So you keep a close eye on the child and respond accordingly. But keep in mind that a healthy child can manifest these symptoms and go through them relatively gracefully and quickly, while the sick child may have a serious response from the expression and need to be hospitalized. The healthy child is free of subluxation, so his body is working optimally and efficiently. The subluxated child is sick and so his nervous system has less control over his body and its ability to respond appropriately. In chiropractic, we believe that by and large, the control of the body should be left to its innate intelligence rather than to a doctor whose sole objective is to suppress all symptoms.

"Modern medicine teaches us to judge all symptoms as bad or wrong, and this is why it seeks to arrest, reduce, and suppress them. Chiropractors don't judge symptoms as bad. We see them as messages and the body's attempts to communicate to us. Let's say you and I ate some bad clams last night, and we were up all night vomiting. Were we sick?"

I saw what he was getting at and answered a vague, "I guess not."

He frowned. "I'd call it healthy, wouldn't you? Our bodies have ingested poison and are wisely removing it. Of course that's a healthy response. I'd say we were sick if we *didn't* throw up all night.

And it's the same with mucous production and fevers to remove and fight bacteria, viruses and other pathogens."

We traveled without speaking for a while. Uncle Earl hummed a tune while I admired the scenery and scanned the deep woods for wildlife.

He broke the silence. "When I was a teenager, I spent some time with my dad in his pediatric office. A father came in once with his three young sons. The oldest boy had chronic tonsillitis and the antibiotics were ineffective, so dad scheduled him for a tonsillectomy. You want to know what my dad said to the father? *Why don't we schedule the other two boys for tonsillectomies at the same time?* The father asked why, since the other two were healthy and had no sore throats or tonsillitis. You know what my dad answered? *Tonsils are vestigial organs and they're better off without them.* Better off without them? Can you believe that? That was the thinking back then. Nature provides us with two huge lymph glands in the back of our throats to act as the body's first line of defense, and doctors told us they were unnecessary. They couldn't have been more wrong. That was 'modern' medicine in the 20th century."

"What did the father of the boys do?"

"Fortunately for the two boys, he said *no thanks* to dad. But I know there were many healthy children that had tonsillectomies back then. How pathetic. How barbaric. Thousands of healthy children were put under anesthesia and had their tonsils surgically removed simply because medical science didn't know what tonsils did. Some died too, either from the anesthesia or from complications like hemorrhage or infection. Healthy kids. In the 1970s, the number of tonsillectomies declined, although it's still a fairly popular surgical procedure to this day, in spite of lots of medical research that says that they are minimally effective or only temporarily beneficial.

"And I know you're aware of myringotomies, when they pierce a hole in the eardrum with a knife or a laser, aren't you. Adam?"

I recalled the pain of ear infections as a boy. "I had that done when I was seven or eight for my ear infections."

"I remember. That brought about one of the many great arguments between your dad and me. Doctors actually told parents – and some *still* do – that the Eustachian tubes were angled too greatly, and that's why the fluid pressure in the ear builds up. So surgery is necessary. Let's cut little holes in the child's eardrum, and insert little grommets because God made a mistake when designing the Eustachian tubes of children. Everything else is amazing and nearly perfect, but the ears need surgical intervention to make things right. Ahh, now the child can be healthy. Does that make any sense to you?"

I just stared at him and smiled meekly.

"Did you know that piercing the eardrum as a medical procedure began in 1649 when a doctor *accidentally* perforated a patient's eardrum while cleaning the ear? The patient's hearing improved and tubes in the ears began. More than 350 years later, we're still doing a lot of them, although like tonsillectomies, their efficacy is questioned by many doctors and researchers."

His face reddened. "You know what I get most angry at? Parents that submit their young children to these barbaric procedures without trying something other than a medical approach. Medical doctors have failed their child for months or years, mostly with antibiotic therapy, but parents stick with them and *then* allow the surgeons to wield their scalpels."

His voice rose. "They submit their child to years of antibiotics and other drugs and questionable and potentially very harmful surgery, and yet they're afraid of a chiropractor because some ignorant person said or wrote that chiropractic might be dangerous for the child. Do you see the insanity here? Kids put under the knife for surgery that may or may not make them any better? And remember; *better*, to them means less symptomatic. It doesn't mean healthier. And although some parents may say that their child is healthier after the tonsillectomy, I doubt it. Obviously, without tonsils you can't have any more tonsillitis, but don't be fooled; that child is not healthier. He's just less symptomatic, at least for the time being. Cutting out tonsils and adenoids and putting tubes in eardrums can't possibly make anyone healthier. Sometimes, simple dietary changes help these kids. Removing dairy and sugar from their diets often makes them healthier, stronger and less acidic and mucous filled.

"Chiropractic has helped thousands of children improve and heal from ear infections, sore throats, tonsillitis and sinus and upper respiratory infections, and saved them from tonsillectomies, adenoidectomies and myringotomies. And yet still many pediatricians don't consider chiropractic an option. Why? Because chiropractors haven't clearly explained to them the logic and safety of what we do. There's so much confusion within the chiropractic profession and so its simple beauty gets lost in the pile of non-chiropractic stuff that so many chiropractors do.

"Research has shown that 85 percent of children in the United States will experience an ear infection before the age of three. My experience has shown me that about 85 percent of kids under regular chiropractic care will not. I know that's a bold statement, but this little town of Southold Springs is living proof. Without a doubt, children are healthier with chiropractic care.

"So, routine tonsillectomies were an experiment that failed. But you must realize that *all* of medicine is an experiment. In the United States, tonsillectomies and myringotomies are done in some regions a lot more than in others. And it has nothing to do with diet or environment. It's just the opinions and judgments of doctors.

Not science. Not proof. Just doctors demonstrating different *opinions* about how to treat people. Our modern system of medicine, namely drugs and surgery, is a giant experiment, and we are all the guinea pigs. All these thousands of man-made pharmaceuticals and surgical procedures are experiments, and mostly failed ones at that. The British Medical Journal recently reported that approximately 2,000 of the 3,000 medical treatments available today are ineffective, unscientific and unproven. Two-thirds! They use the guise of science to justify them, but there's little to no real science when it comes to drugs and surgery. They are simply the best medicine has to offer at this point in time."

I started to speak, but he kept going.

"I know, what about life-saving appendectomies and cancer surgeries? Yes, many surgeries save lives. And don't forget trauma medicine. It's absolutely wonderful how these men and women save lives every day. But we're not talking about that. We're talking about the consciousness, the science, or more accurately, the *illusion* of science, and the day-to-day health care of millions of people. I truly believe that 100 years from now, we'll look back at today's modern medicine and roll our eyes in disbelief. Just like looking back 100 years ago from today. We squirm when we hear some of the things medicine did in 1915.

"Our pharmaceutically driven modern medicine is actually in its infancy. It's only been around for about 60 to 70 years. I understand the attempt to develop and use chemicals to affect the function of the body and mind. But as this experiment in chemistry progresses, it should become safer, and yet it doesn't appear to be. More than 200 million Americans take at least one medicine daily, and more than 150 million take two or more daily. If pharmaceutical companies' sales keep escalating at the rate they have in the past 20 years, every man, woman and child in America will be on multiple daily medications in the near future. And every child will receive between 100 and 200 vaccines before kindergarten. Scary stuff.

"And for all the good modern medicine does, it still manages to do a lot of harm. Medical mistakes and prescription drugs have become two of the major causes of death in this country, and yet very few people seem to question it. In their defense, medical practitioners deal with the majority of the population, very *sick* people, very *old* people, very *subluxated* people, and life and death situations daily. But there's no doubt that they need to be more conservative and conscious with their care, and treat the body with more love, respect and reverence. And even more importantly, they need to know that chiropractic is a safe, sound and viable necessity for people." He added, "Ironically, chiropractic adheres to the great medical creed, *first do no harm*, while modern medicine does not.

"This is why I say that we must *think*. But the drug companies and medical community don't want you to question them. They prefer you to be sheep and do what you are told. Get your shots. Take your medicine. *They* are the authorities and only *they* know what's best for you."

I thought of my father and spoke up. "I don't mean to sound disrespectful Uncle Earl, but sometimes you sound really radical. And they *are* the authorities, aren't they?"

"As you heard me say to the group last night, please feel free to challenge my logic and my thinking, Adam. I welcome all questions, and don't worry about seeming disrespectful. Speak your mind. As far as being the authority, chiropractors study the same human body as medical doctors do, often using the same textbooks. Chiropractic cadaver labs are no different than those of medical students. So, I'll gladly admit that medical doctors are the authorities on drugs and surgery, as well as emergency and disease care, but I believe they fall way short when it comes to health. They are so busy controlling and suppressing symptoms with drugs that they've lost sight of what health actually is, and therefore, they are *not* the authority on health."

"I guess chiropractic is just so new to me. That's why it sounds extreme sometimes."

He laughed gently. "It *is* new to you, Adam. You, as well as most of the millions born in this country in the past 50 years or so have been born and raised in a medicine cabinet. Any other way of thinking is foreign and heretical. Have I said anything that's not true or reasonable?"

My mind reeled with all this new information, but I mumbled, "No. I don't think so."

"I know I sound like a radical sometimes, but it's just that I take time to *think*. That's one of the reasons I love to kayak in the stillness of the lake. So many people drive to work with the radio on listening to music, sports, news or politics, do their job at work, drive home again with the radio on again, eat, watch TV, and go to bed. During many of those hours, they are bombarded with drug commercials. They are numbed with television, sports, shopping, drugs, alcohol, gambling, sex and stress. They accept what's in the news or on the Internet. They accept what they've been told since childhood – *Don't go outside without a jacket, you'll catch cold. Breakfast is the most important meal of the day.* They rarely question *anything* because they've been taught not to question the teacher, preacher or doctor. That's why I say that we are becoming a nation of sheep, and of course to them, a lot of what I say sounds weird, extreme or radical. Actually, what I offer is much more conservative than drugs and surgery, not to mention safer, simpler and more logical. Today's health care, namely vaccines, drugs and surgeries, is what's really radical and extreme. We've just come to accept them as normal due to our medical indoctrination.

"But am I trying to convince people to think like me? No, I'm just trying to open their minds and get them to think, *period*. And I'm not trying to replace their medical way of thinking, but rather add to it by teaching the importance of the spine and nervous system and their relationship to health. There's no doubt in my mind that if people changed nothing else in their lifestyles but the addition of regular chiropractic care, they would be much healthier. The difference would be night and day. I also remind people that within them lies a great power to heal, a simple truth forgotten or ignored by modern medicine.

"Drug companies used to spend more on research and development than on marketing. Not anymore. More money now goes into marketing than research. Why? Why do drug companies spend more on marketing than just about any other organization on earth? Because it works, and because they don't want you to think. They want to do your thinking for you. That's what marketing is all about – get peoples' thought processes aligned with their products, and they'll never have to think again. So we end up with people that walk up and down the drug store aisles and buy this for their sinuses, this for their acne, this for their scratchy throat, this for their indigestion, and this for their hemorrhoids. These people never question or think for a moment that what they're doing is counterproductive to their health and counterproductive to living better lives. They rarely, if ever, consider that putting all these poisonous chemicals into their bodies on a daily basis might actually be diminishing their health, reducing their quality of life, and shortening their lives. To them, it's normal. To me, it's insanity."

"So you don't take any medicines at all?"

"Every now and then I buy some herbal cough drops, but that's about it. You may have noticed that I sometimes talk a bit. I took an antibiotic for two weeks about 10 years ago when a tick bit me and caused the Lyme's bull's-eye rash on my shoulder. I weighed the value and risk of taking the antibiotic versus the risk of getting Lyme's disease, and decided to take the antibiotic. But I'm talking about the *daily* intake of these poisons to suppress or alleviate symptoms that are usually the body's attempt to express or communicate."

"So you're saying it's wrong for people to take medicine?"

"No. I'm not a medical doctor and I *never* tell people *not* to take medicine, or take less or more or something else instead. I'm sure there are actual times when people really need and benefit from medicine, and it's not my place to determine those times. I do think that as a society, however, we take *way* too much medicine, and I think the consciousness of the nation has become brainwashed into drug dependency. And *that* I believe is wrong when health is the objective."

"You called them poisons. You believe that?"

"Yes. They *are* poisons. When you ingest these drugs, whether prescription or over the counter, do you think your body responds with, *thank goodness this drug just came in. Now we can be healthier?* It doesn't. It sees the drug as a foreign poison and tries to detoxify and eliminate it through any means possible. During the process of the body rejecting the drug, the drug *might* give the person the desired effect." He paused and continued, "An old ad for constipation medicine used to say, *this medicine will move your bowels,* but it's actually the opposite that happens; the bowels move the medicine. The bowels move the medicine outward because it's poison. But keep in mind that they are *all* poisons. Hey, if they were good for us, shouldn't we *all* take them?

"One of my big questions regarding taking medicine has always been, *does it make you healthier?* It's very rare when a drug does that. I've walked the huge aisles of the pharmacies, and I haven't found a medicine that actually makes people healthier. Hey, if taking a medicine made someone healthy, then those who take lots of medicines should be the healthiest people."

I interjected, "But what about insulin for a diabetic?"

"I guess you got me there, Adam. That's a replacement drug, which means it's replacing insulin that's not being produced by the individual's pancreas. I think we've got to back up a step and ask why the pancreas stopped producing insulin in the first place. There are many factors, but often, the pancreas is probably just overloaded by years of excessive sugar ingestion. But follow my thinking here; if your pancreas stops functioning properly, meaning it isn't producing the proper amounts of insulin at the right times, you are not healthy. Substituting with an artificial or external source of insulin doesn't make you healthy. It makes you survive, which is a good thing, but it doesn't make you healthy. Do you see the difference?"

"But that artificial insulin allows you to live."

"True. But health means function. It doesn't just mean living. So I would say that these drugs are certainly beneficial and life-saving for diabetics, but they don't actually make them healthier. They regulate blood sugar levels, but they don't improve the way the body functions."

I couldn't believe what I was hearing, and surprised myself when I angrily and loudly asked, "How can you say that about medicine? And how can you compare medicine to chiropractic? Medicine is huge and it saves countless lives every day."

He smiled warmly at me. "Yes it does, Adam. I'd never argue that. And I'm not comparing medicine to chiropractic. I'm aware that there are many life-saving drugs and procedures out there. I'm not *anti*-medicine; I'm *pro*-health. It's absolutely pointless to argue the virtues of medicine versus chiropractic or herbalism or homeopathy or anything else. Every person has a unique state of awareness, and each chooses his or her own path of healing. As far as I see, there *is* no comparison, but if you like, we'll compare before the end of the weekend. The main reason I go after medicine sometimes is because I believe the medical profession doesn't want people to think and because I disagree strongly with its attempt – and overall success – at becoming a monopoly in health care.

"Let me tell you a story about a man with whom I went to chiropractic college. His name was Bobby. He was a diabetic, and at age 29, the diabetes medicine he'd taken for seven years was not working anymore. His blood sugar was out of control, his entire body was swollen and dark purple, he was in constant agony, and his medical doctors told him he would die in less than a month. Bobby went to visit his dad to say his goodbyes, and his dad took him immediately to his chiropractor. After two weeks of daily adjustments, Bobby's pancreas came back to life and he became healthy. He could eat and drink anything he liked, just like you and I. When he went back to his medical doctors a few months later, robust and healthy, they were dumbfounded. They demanded to know about the miraculous treatment that saved him. When Bobby told them he went to a chiropractor, they mocked him and told him he was granted a wonderful gift from nature, and that the chiropractor had nothing to do with it."

He drank some water and continued. "When people think a certain way, it's very difficult for them to consider another viewpoint. Without any real understanding of chiropractic, many in medicine are quick to ridicule or reject it. This only contributes to medicine's dangerous monopoly of health care." He paused and added, "But little did those doctors know that the wonderful gift from nature *is* chiropractic."

"During the Revolutionary War, when our founding fathers were designing our new and free country, Dr. Benjamin Rush, at the Constitutional Convention said, *the Constitution of this Republic should make special provision for medical freedom. To restrict the art of healing to one class will constitute the Bastille of medical science. All such laws are un-American and despotic. Unless we put medical freedom into the constitution the time will come when medicine will organize into an undercover dictatorship and force people who wish doctors and treatment of their own choice to submit to only what the dictating outfit offers."*

He sighed and added, "One main reason medicine organized and formed the AMA in 1845 was to oppress and obliterate homeopathy, the largest alternative to medicine at that time. Similarly, they tried their best to eliminate chiropractic in the 20th century. For decades, B.J. Palmer used to tell the medical community that if they really wanted to get rid of chiropractic, all they had to do was get sick people well." We shared a laugh at this. "But seriously, they don't like competition, and I've always felt that when the objective is a healthier society, cooperation is far greater than competition in the healing arts. Fortunately, chiropractic and homeopathy survived, but most people still don't know what either does. To this day, medicine still perpetuates the myth that they *alone* are rooted in science, while chiropractic, homeopathy, and everything else that isn't part of the medical world, is not.

"They also tried to destroy osteopathy, but osteopathy succumbed to their pressure and chose to join medicine rather than oppose it. In the U.S. today, a doctor of osteopathy, or D.O., can do anything a medical doctor can do. A D.O. can be an internist, a cardiologist, an obstetrician or a surgeon. And you know what they say about two things being exactly the same, don't you? One of them is unnecessary."

I had looked into schools of Osteopathic Medicine, so I quickly said, "Some osteopaths perform manipulation, and so they *are* different from M.D.s."

He smiled at my boldness. "True Adam, but M.D.s can manipulate too if they choose. And it's a very small percentage of osteopaths that manipulate. I've met a few D.O.s that grin condescendingly when referring to manipulation. One told me that it was an elective course when he was in school, and that most of the students chose to ignore or reject it. Why? I believe because the basic premise of osteopathy was weak and flawed, and that's why it didn't really survive. In the late 1800s, both osteopathy and chiropractic were discovered. Chiropractic focused on specific adjustments to the spine to free the nervous system, while osteopathy used general manipulation to promote health and improve circulation.

"I find it very interesting that osteopaths originally knew that manipulating the spine helped people, but due to their weak philosophy and general manipulation skills and techniques, they didn't get the results that chiropractors have gotten for 120 years. Chiropractic endured almost a century of tremendous medical oppression, yet survived because its basic premises are sound and logical, and mostly because it helped, and continues to help, millions of people live healthier and richer lives. It saddens me that there are some in chiropractic that would rather abandon chiropractic's principles and follow the path of osteopathy and join medicine. That's why it's important to me that chiropractors keep their own language. I cringe when I hear chiropractors use words like manipulation, spinal manipulative therapy or treatment. It's an *adjustment*, a chiropractic *adjustment*.

"There is so much confusion within the chiropractic profession today, not due to a flawed philosophy, but rather because so many chiropractors have never been taught our basic philosophy. They've grown up in the medical, symptom-treating paradigm and believe chiropractic to be a part of that. In school, they are taught to become lower back and neck pain treaters. To diagnose and refer.

To think of themselves as primary portals of health care that know when and where to properly refer people."

I interrupted, "Primary portals of health care?"

"Yes. Some chiropractors think they can diagnose like the M.D. because they studied diagnosis. But they haven't endured the rigors of medical internships and residencies. If you had a serious cough or respiratory problem, which would you rather see? A chiropractor who has studied lung sounds in a textbook, or a medical doctor who not only studied them in a textbook, but was also taught from a qualified doctor, and has listened to – *experienced* – the various lung sounds? He's actually *heard* patients with pneumonia, pleurisy, COPD and bronchitis."

I smiled and said, "It sounds like you're promoting medicine now."

He smiled back at me and said, "I respect them very much for their dedication and skills. But life is a lot easier when you know who you are. I know what it is to be a chiropractor that doesn't try to be like a medical doctor. And chiropractic, in this simple chiropractor's opinion, is at its very best when it is non-diagnostic, non-therapeutic, and not trying to be an alternative or substitute for medicine.

"The basic principles of chiropractic are not taught in our chiropractic colleges, so many newly trained chiropractors graduate with an identity problem. They're not M.D.s, simply because they haven't earned that degree, and they're not principled chiropractors, so they haven't got the basic idea of correcting subluxations to improve the integrity of the human nervous system. Instead, they are lost somewhere in between, so they end up being spinal manipulators to give relief to people with back pain and headaches. Their offices are usually easy to spot. Their advertising and language are about relief from back and neck pain, most of their patients are there for pain relief, and they rarely adjust children. Although they may fill a need in society, they're missing out on the greater picture of subluxation correction. They are missing what B.J. Palmer called *The Big Idea.*

"I strongly believe that if we took a small percentage of the money we use for medical research and put it into chiropractic, herbal and homeopathic research, we'd find that the population would be much healthier and the cost of health care in this country would be a fraction of what it is today. Medicine will always be the bastion of emergency and trauma care, as well as advanced disease care. But regarding the general health of the population, it falls short. Way short. As long as they keep thinking all the answers lie in chemistry, namely vaccines and pharmaceuticals, they are off target.

"And speaking of off target, when a medical doctor of any kind, nurse, PA or PT tells a patient *not* to go to a chiropractor for any reason whatsoever, that person is showing his or her ignorance. Sometimes the reason is simply because chiropractic is not part of their medical team. But often, it's part of the leftover malice and attempt to discredit chiropractic. They may say that chiropractic is dangerous for children or for someone who's had a stroke, or that chiropractic can't help you because you have this disease or condition. All untrue. All signs of ignorance and bias. I suggest you find a new doctor, PA or PT, one with a more open-minded understanding of health and healing.

"My mission in life is to teach chiropractic as simply as possible, and to as many as possible. Some will grasp its beauty and simplicity, and some will reject it intensely. Interestingly though, most of those who oppose chiropractic the most powerfully have never experienced it. And when asked what they actually *know* about chiropractic, the answer is usually, *nothing.* They just don't like us because we're not part of their familiar medical paradigm. I agree with Thomas Jefferson when he said that one of our worst failings as human beings is *condemnation without investigation.* That said, let's give you the experience of a chiropractic adjustment."

We pulled into town and turned into the office parking lot. It was busier than when I was there yesterday.

Education is not the learning of facts,
but the training of the mind to think.

Albert Einstein

10

As we got out of Uncle Earl's Jeep, a tall, muscular man in an army uniform walked towards us and yelled out a powerful, "Hello Doctor Earl." Uncle Earl introduced me to Harry and asked him to tell me his story.

Harry stood about six feet, six inches tall and smiled from ear to ear as he looked me in the eye and shook my hand. "I'd be happy to, sir. When I was 14, I was diagnosed with scoliosis and told I needed surgery after exercises, physical therapy and braces failed. I don't know if you know about scoliosis surgery, but they insert a metal rod in your spine and then fuse the entire spine from top to bottom. You're in a full body cast for months and the rehab is long and arduous. Well, luckily for me, my parents decided to try chiropractic three weeks before my scheduled surgery. Dr. Earl adjusted my spine and during the next few weeks and months, it got straighter and straighter. I grew almost a foot in about a year, and never needed the surgery. Thank God, because I never would've gotten into the army and been able to serve and enjoy life like I do." He put his arm around Uncle Earl's shoulder. "Thanks, Dr. Earl. Nice meeting you, Adam," and he walked on.

Uncle Earl turned to me. "Do you know how many of these scoliosis surgeries are done on little boys and girls each year? Yes, sometimes they're absolutely necessary to avoid future damage to organs and glands, but I've seen the pre-surgical x-rays of some of these kids and I think these doctors should be put in jail for not at least trying chiropractic before they surgically alter these kids' lives forever."

"Jail?" I asked, surprised at his statement.

"Yes, jail. Although they are ignorant of what we do, it's still criminal, when simple, safe chiropractic adjustments can improve the spines of a great number of these children. Braces, exercises and physical therapy usually fail these kids because they don't address the subluxations. And when these fail to have a positive impact on the curvatures of the spine, the next step is surgery. The parents of some of these kids need to have their heads examined too. Or more kindly put, expand their awareness. If a doctor recommended such drastic and invasive surgery for one of my children, I'd investigate *every* reasonable option available."

We walked into the large waiting room. In it were more than 30 people, including about a dozen infants and children. A young, blonde girl ran up and hugged Uncle Earl the moment we walked in and I thought that was pretty cool. I'd only seen that a few times in 20 years while I was in my dad's office. Among the many colorful paintings and posters on the walls were obvious messages of chiropractic, including the words *life, power, ease, subluxation, love, adjustment and innate intelligence*. A large banner across the entire front wall read, *Chiropractic Saves Lives*, and I smiled inwardly, thinking about our last few minutes in the car.

Uncle Earl greeted the women at the front desk and a few other patients. We walked through a door and into a hallway that led to five rooms, two on the left, two on the right, and one at the end of the hall. The first two rooms had three adjusting tables in each, and the second two had two in each. I saw my cousin Megan in one and she came over quickly and gave me a strong hug. We exchanged greetings, but she was busy adjusting, so Uncle Earl grabbed my arm gently and led me to the room at the end of the hallway. In it were a desk, three chairs and one adjusting table. I noticed x-rays in a viewing box near the desk. Above the table was a small poster on the wall that read, *I Adjust This Spine with All My Love*. Another banner above us read, *Your Spine – The Key to Health*.

"Hop on," boomed Uncle Earl in a loving way. "Let's give you an adjustment."

I laid face down on the table. "I'm just confirming what I mentioned earlier, Adam. The rotation of the pelvis and the subluxations of the upper cervical spine." He examined my leg length and moved my legs up and down. He ran his hands up and down my spine, lightly at first, then a bit firmer. He then asked me to turn my head left and right. He placed some wedges under my pelvis and asked me to take a few deep breaths while he pressed down gently on my pelvis. Then he asked me to lie on my right side so he could move my left sacroiliac joint. He gently used my leg as a lever and I felt a little crack. It felt good. Next, he easily adjusted my neck, and I heard a few more pops.

"Okay, Adam. That's it for now. There's more life in your body, and your body and mind are improving at this very moment."

It was less than three minutes. "That's it?" I asked, surprised. "All these years of fear and apprehension about a chiropractic adjustment, and it was a piece of cake that only took a minute or two."

He smiled and said, "It's not how much we do, but *what* we do that matters. To someone who's been in a dark room for years, the click of a light switch makes a huge difference."

I mentioned the times I heard dad and a few other doctors talk about the dangers of a chiropractic adjustment. "But why would they say that to people, Uncle Earl. It's not really dangerous at all, is it?"

"Shouldn't you have asked me that *before* you got adjusted?" We both laughed. "Actually, chiropractic is very safe. And not only is it safe, but it's probably the simplest way available to improve your health. For what you put into it, five to ten minutes on a table, you get so much out of it. There's no doubt in my mind that you truly are healthier with each adjustment.

"Regarding safety, insurance companies don't deal with rumor and innuendo, Adam. They deal with facts and statistics. And the fact is that a chiropractor's malpractice premiums are a fraction of medical doctors'. The reason? Chiropractors don't hurt people, but drugs and surgeries do."

"But I read online last night that chiropractic is just a theory and that it could be dangerous, especially if it keeps people from seeking proper medical treatment."

Uncle Earl smiled at that. "We'll talk about *proper medical treatment* later. As far as chiropractic being a theory, that's nonsense. Wait here a moment." He walked out of the room and came back about two minutes later with a heavy-set young woman and a small and very chubby boy.

"Please sit," said Uncle Earl. "Nancy, this is my nephew, Adam. Adam, this is Nancy and her two-year-old son, Angelo. Thank you Nancy, for sharing your story. Please tell Adam about little Angelo."

Nancy spoke quickly. "When Angelo was born, he couldn't breathe too well. With every breath, he sounded like this…" and she made a weird, deep and gravely rumble with her throat. "He spent his first three weeks in the neonatal intensive care unit, and had six specialists examine him. They couldn't figure out what was wrong with him. After that time and many different medicines and treatments, he was no better, so they told my husband and me to take him home. One doctor told us there's a good chance he could die in the next few weeks, and to be prepared just in case. Every night his breathing got worse. This went on for months. I rarely slept and neither did my husband. Well, my husband finally got so stressed out that he left us when Angelo was four months old. I haven't seen or heard from him since. Right after Angelo's seven-month birthday, someone told me I should drive him to Southold Springs to see Dr. Hale." She paused to compose herself, but appeared to be on the verge of tears. "After his very first adjustment, his breathing was about 50 percent better that night. And after his second adjustment the very next day, he breathed quietly and normally like a little boy should." She started to cry while thanking and hugging Uncle Earl. He handed her a tissue and thanked her again for sharing her story. I thanked her too, and she and Angelo walked out of the room.

Uncle Earl looked serious and asked, "And you ask if chiropractic is a theory? Would you like to ask Nancy if she thinks chiropractic is a theory? Do you think it matters to her what the Internet says about chiropractic? How about Harry? Would he have been better off following *proper* medical treatment? And there are thousands of similar stories in chiropractic offices around the world today. Eye problems, asthma, colic, constipation, bedwetting, allergies, ear infections. Infants and children respond to chiropractic amazingly well. And *that's* why I think it's tragic that half the chiropractors are treating adults with backaches and neck pain. In their hands, they hold a special gift to help a very sick society. They have the capacity to help infants and children lead healthier and more productive lives, and instead they spend their days treating and *manipulating* low backs to ease pain." He cringed when he said the word *manipulating,* and added, "Who wants to be *manipulated*? I don't. Manipulation implies control. Chiropractors *adjust*. We make *adjustments* to the spine. It's a freeing process. We don't try to control *anything* in the body because we trust that the subluxation-free body knows what it's doing.

"Did you notice the little blond girl who hugged me in the waiting room? Her name is Emma and she's five years old. When she was born, her right eye was completely turned inward. You couldn't see the iris at all, just the white. The parents were told she needed *at least* two surgeries to repair the eye, but they said it would be best to wait until she was three months old. At two months, they brought her in to see me. I'd never seen anything quite like that before, but when I checked her spine, sure enough, her atlas was subluxated to the right. I adjusted her, and within a few seconds, the eyeball turned to center. The next morning, the eye had turned inward again. I adjusted her again, and the eyeball straightened out, this time for three days. After her third adjustment, the eye stayed centered. She never needed surgery and her vision is perfect. Now how many people would ever consider a chiropractor for a situation like that? Fortunately for Emma, her parents did.

"In the 1940s, a famous medical doctor's wife was very sick for many months. Dozens of doctors ordered dozens of tests and tried various medicines and treatments, but the doctor's wife continued to get sicker and weaker. As a last resort, this doctor boldly drove his wife from Minnesota to see Dr. B.J. Palmer in Davenport, Iowa. The doctor brought in stacks of records, x-rays and lab work. When B.J. declined to even *look* at all the woman's medical information, the doctor called him ignorant. B.J. reminded the doctor that all these tests and procedures had not helped his wife get well, and therefore *he* was the one who was ignorant, especially of the spine's and nervous system's role in health. B.J. x-rayed and adjusted the woman's upper cervical spine, and in a few weeks, she was healthy and strong."

We went upstairs and I greeted my aunt Cathy again. Aware that I was leaving for home tomorrow, she said, "After dinner, you and Earl can talk some more and then we'll all go watch the fireworks. How's that sound to you, Adam?"

"Great, aunt Cathy," I said. "Thank you."

Uncle Earl made fresh-squeezed orange juice and we sat on two lounge chairs on a large upstairs deck. The view of the mountains was spectacular.

"So what do you say about proper medical treatment for Harry, Emma and Angelo?" he asked with a touch of sarcasm.

I let out a big sigh and shrugged my shoulders.

"Exactly. There's not much *to* say. I could tell you a dozen stories of chiropractors who've gone into hospitals to adjust an infant whose parents were told that the child would likely die in a day or two. And guess what? The babies miraculously came back to life. After one or two adjustments. Now certainly medicine saves some of these babies, and some they don't save, and their deaths are labeled as crib death, SIDS or something similar. But the bigger point is that chiropractic should be available to every newborn. Every baby and child should be checked for subluxations. The wise medical doctor should strongly recommend to every parent to make sure each child is examined and adjusted by a chiropractor. Unfortunately for the health of our nation, we're probably a long way from that. Like so many others, Angelo's problem was not in his lungs or bronchi, but in the nerve supply *to* his lungs and bronchi." He paused a moment, then added, "And Emma? I don't know the precise mechanism of how a little atlas subluxation can cause the eye musculature to malfunction. But it did. It somehow affected the cranial nerve supply to the muscles of the eyeball."

He sipped some juice. "Chiropractic is no more a theory than medicine is a theory. Just because you see a lot of *sciencey*-looking people in white lab coats wearing stethoscopes and surgical masks doesn't make medicine a science. And just because some ignorant person on television or the Internet says, *there's no scientific evidence to support the theory of chiropractic*, doesn't make chiropractic unscientific. There's tons of evidence, and there are thousands of stories like Angelo's and Emma's out there. Our culture is just brainwashed into thinking a certain way. When medically-oriented people repeat something enough, it's generally blindly accepted as truth. So the public ends up believing that medicine is based on real science while chiropractic, homeopathy, herbalism and acupuncture get lumped into the unscientific fringe element with crystals and faith healing."

He got up, grabbed a notebook that was on a table inside, and sat down again. He opened the notebook. "Marcia Angell, M.D., a former editor-in-chief at the *New England Journal of Medicine* said, 'it is simply no longer possible to believe much of the clinical research that is published, or to rely on the judgment of trusted physicians or authoritative medical guidelines. I take no pleasure in this conclusion, which I reached slowly and reluctantly over my two decades as editor of *The New England Journal of Medicine*.'

"Referring to our current American medical model of health care, she stated in a PBS interview, 'if we had set out to design the worst system that we could imagine, we couldn't have imagined one as bad as we have.' In the same interview, she urged the nation to 'scrap its failing healthcare system and start over.'"

He smiled and added, "There's no doubt we have to change the way we do things, but we first need to change the way we *think*. We need to get rid of drug commercials on TV, and we need to stop the incessant brainwashing of our culture into sickness and disease. The word *cancer* alone is forced into our minds many times daily. Contrary to popular belief, we *don't* need to increase our awareness of breast cancer, Parkinson's and Alzheimer's. We need to increase our awareness of *health*. We are never going to be a healthy society until we start *thinking* healthy. We need to teach our children to place their trust and confidence in their magnificent bodies and the power that created them. *Then* we can change our approach and application regarding health. And that means chiropractic care for everyone." He paused and then added, "But what a brave woman. It's not easy going up against the medical establishment. Some have lost their licenses for such heresy.

"We want to believe that all doctors are good, and everything they prescribe must be good for us as well. And the pharmaceutical companies, too. They truly have the public's best interest at heart, don't they? I can't help but think that medicine is on a bad path and heading in the wrong direction. More vaccines, more drugs and more surgeries are not the way to better health, and the U.S. is shining proof of that. When something doesn't work, *more* of it will not magically turn it into something that works.

"Medical care is becoming more business-oriented by the day. Hospitals and corporations are currently buying doctors' offices for one reason – to control where the money goes. As more hospital boards and administrators push to fill their beds with patients to increase profits, our society suffers. The goal should be to have *fewer* people in hospitals, not more. It is truly bad medicine. Good business, but bad medicine.

"This is why I speak of objectives. The medical objective is to treat and conquer disease. The chiropractic objective is to improve human performance by the correction of vertebral subluxation. Health is the natural by-product of optimum performance.

"Is medicine a science? Partly. But it's mostly an art. If it was a pure and true science, such as mathematics, astronomy, or chemistry *in a lab*, you would be treated exactly the same by every doctor, not just in this country, but around the world as well. Heck, doctors on the same street don't treat the same case identically. One will recommend drug A, another will recommend drugs B and C, and a third will recommend surgery. That's not science.

"Don't get me wrong, there's lots of science in the *technology* in medicine. Lab and blood tests, X-rays, CTs, MRIs, ultrasound, PETscans, and so on. These are amazing demonstrations of science. Laboratories use science to analyze blood and tissues, and to diagnose conditions and diseases. But when it comes to treatment, the science is questionable at best. When doctors prescribe drugs or perform surgery on the human body, it's more art than science. It's really, *this is what we think is best right now*, and that is not science. The *illusion* of science is there, but the *actual* science, no.

"Real science is reproducible time and again. Mathematics is pure science. Two plus two is four in Colorado, in Japan, and on the moon. Always. Astronomy is a science that can tell us to the minute when the next full moon will appear in the sky, or when the next solar eclipse will occur. Chemistry in a laboratory is a science. Combine sodium and chloride, and providing all other qualifying factors are equal, you'll get sodium chloride – salt – every single time. But chemistry in the living human body is not a science. It *cannot* tell us precisely what an individual's response to taking something as simple as an aspirin will be, let alone the thousands of other drugs on the market. Even simple acetaminophen – Tylenol – has been linked to asthma in children, not to mention a leading cause of liver failure. And what about people taking multiple medicines? I've met some folks that take 18 prescriptions a day! No one, not the greatest doctor, scientist, chemist or pharmacist in the world knows what these combined chemicals do inside an individual's body and mind. This becomes a guessing or percentage game at best. There are too many variables, and the biggest of these is the uniqueness of every individual state of consciousness. And we're all aware that taking one medicine often leads to the need for other medicines to counteract the ill effects of the first one."

"Well, what kind of science is there in chiropractic?"

"Very simple. Your nervous system controls and coordinates all parts of the body. Fact. Vertebral subluxations interfere with that nervous system's transmission, altering its coordination and control over the body, creating a weakened or dis-eased body. Fact. Correct the subluxation and you improve the nervous system's ability to function properly, which allows the harmonious communication and function of the entire body and mind. Logical conclusion.

He continued. "If I tightly wrap a rubber band around your aorta, the large artery exiting the heart, do you need science and double-blind studies to tell you that a tight rubber band around the aorta is bad for the body? Of course not. Do you want to treat the symptoms that the rubber band would likely cause, like high blood pressure? You could, but wouldn't it be wiser to simply remove the rubber band?

"Does vertebral subluxation interfere with the function of the nervous system? You bet. Always. And it *always* results in weakness and dis-ease, regardless of our inability to qualify and quantify that weakness. Every subluxation causes this, regardless of the presence or absence of pain or symptoms. Although medical science doesn't fully understand the concept or the devastating effects of vertebral subluxation, for 100 years they have certainly proven that changes in the position and/or mobility of vertebrae alter nerve function. One study from the University of Colorado showed that the weight of a dime on a nerve root diminishes that nerves ability to function properly.

"In the September, 2005 issue of *Spine*, one of the scientific community's most prestigious orthopedic journals, there was a paper presented by six medical doctors regarding the relationship between forward head carriage and general health. Now keep in mind, forward head carriage is but *one of many* common types of vertebral subluxation. They examined and x-rayed 752 adults, and measured the degree of forward head carriage as well as general health status indicators such as heart, lungs, digestion, energy level and immune function. Here's what they discovered:

One – There was a deterioration of health status with forward head carriage.

Two – All measures of health status showed significantly poorer scores with forward head carriage.

Three – Even minor forward head carriage is detrimental.

Four – The severity of symptoms increased linearly with progressive increase in forward head carriage.

Five – There was clear evidence of increased pain and decreased function as the degree of forward head carriage increased.

"Unintentionally, they validated what chiropractors have been saying for more than a 100 years; that there is a direct relationship between structure and function in the human body. Traumatic and stressful changes to the spine weaken the body and mind on all levels. Immune function and energy are diminished, organs and glands work less efficiently, and the person's health and life are simply worse. And as insightful as this study is, it means little or nothing to most of medicine. Medical researchers *discover* a basic and profound truth – that the condition of the spine is directly related to the health of the individual – and yet they do absolutely nothing about it. Why? Because there are no drugs that make the spine function better."

I questioned, somewhat angrily, "But why *doesn't* medicine do anything about this?"

Uncle Earl smiled wryly, "Medicine keeps its focus on drugs and surgery. Research of a structural/functional nature gets buried away, ignored and forgotten. Although there are branches of medicine that study structure, they, like many chiropractors, see patients years down the road, *after the fact*. It's not easy to improve the spine of a 65-year-old that's been subluxated for more than 50 years. He can certainly be helped, but it makes much more sense to examine and adjust the spines of infants and children to avoid a lifetime of weakness and all the physical, emotional and mental problems caused by subluxation.

"A medical doctor, F. Batmanghelidj, has written and published papers and a wonderful book, *Your Body's Many Cries for Water*. For more than 20 years, he's been working diligently to get modern medicine to grasp his fundamental principle – that chronic dehydration is responsible for many of today's diseases. Although he's part of the medical world, medicine ignores and rejects his research primarily because the pharmaceutical companies have nothing to gain by people drinking more water.

"So if you're waiting for medicine to prove *chiropractic's* validity, and pat all the chiropractors on the back for doing such a fine job, you're probably going to wait a long time. Remember, there's no money in health, and there's no money given to research a profession that doesn't prescribe drugs. *One* medical school in the U.S. receives more federal money *in one year* for research than the *entire chiropractic profession* has received in more than 100 years. There's your dangerous medical monopoly. He smiled warmly and asked, "Have you had enough of your old uncle's ramblings yet?"

"No. I'm enjoying it. But I realize, like you said, that I *have* been raised in a medicine cabinet. Our family takes medicine for everything. It really is a way of life for us. In the past few years alone, I've taken allergy, skin, cold, sinus, anti-inflammatory, constipation *and* diarrhea medication. And my 24-year-old brother takes heartburn, headache and pain medication every day. I'm starting to question a lot of the comparisons between medicine and chiropractic."

"I tell you this, Adam. It's foolish to compare medicine and chiropractic. Why? Apples and oranges. They are different in every way – in their philosophy, their objective and their application. Chiropractic is neither a substitute nor alternative to medicine or anything else. If someone has a child with asthma, and asks me if he should take the child to a chiropractor *or* a medical doctor, I ask him what he wants to accomplish. *What's your objective?* If the objective is to treat, manage or control the asthma, then I'd say go to a medical doctor. If the objective is health and optimum function, then seek out a chiropractor.

"This is about chiropractic at its very best. Don't ask me whether he should go to a medical doctor *or* a chiropractor. I believe every child should have his spine examined regularly by a chiropractor, and if necessary adjusted, whether he has asthma or not. If a child *has* asthma, he should *certainly* be checked by a chiropractor. My God, asthma is a neurological phenomenon. Of course he should be adjusted. But *instead* of medicine? Never. This is partly why chiropractors were so persecuted in the first half of the 20th century. Although I admire their boldness when they recommended people to go to a chiropractor *instead* of a medical doctor, I think when they did that, they were practicing medicine, which they have no right to do. They were making a judgment regarding the child's need for medical care, and I believe they are not qualified, and therefore wrong for doing that." His voice rose. "This is why chiropractic does not belong in the medical model. Every person, under every circumstance, functions better with a healthier, subluxation-free spine and nervous system. *Period.*

"But since you want to compare, let's compare. Let's take a nine-year-old boy who goes to a medical doctor with a breathing problem? He is given the diagnosis of asthma, given a prescription or two or three, and takes them for the rest of his life. He calls and considers himself an asthmatic for his entire life. Essentially, he is weakened for life. Sad, but all too often, true. And he is weakened in two ways; first, he is weakened by the daily intake of harmful chemicals, the medicine. And second, ignoring subluxations and doing nothing to improve the function of the body weaken him more each day.

"Let's have the same child go to a chiropractor. He gets adjusted, his breathing improves, often dramatically, and he is healthier for life. No label, no diagnosis, no weakness. And no lifetime dependency on drugs. I'd say that's a big difference. There's your comparison. And I'm certainly not foolish enough to say this is the case with every asthmatic child, but my experience has shown that more than 80 percent of these kids will heal and no longer be asthmatic under chiropractic care."

I was amazed. "Why isn't this investigated with huge studies? Do you know how many asthmatics there are in this country?"

Uncle Earl said, "Didn't we just go over that? Welcome to the challenging world of trying to get people to understand a simple principle regarding the state and tone of their central nervous systems and their health. And yes, there are tens of millions of asthmatics in the United States. Thousands die from it every year, and the number of asthmatics grows significantly every single year. How's that for medical success?" He paused and added sarcastically, "Well, asthma *does* keep a lot of doctors, clinics and hospital emergency rooms in business, if you want to call that success."

I thought of the many asthmatics in my dad's office over the years and understood his sarcasm.

He continued. "And the saddest facts are that they, the medical community, never consider asthma a neurological problem, and don't know that chiropractic could help a huge percentage of these people heal from asthma. *Heal*, Adam. Not just control or manage their symptoms for a lifetime, but actually heal from the bloody disease. Instead, they'll often frown condescendingly and tell parents something like, *chiropractic for asthma? Ridiculous.*" His voice rose. "And here's what medicine did to chiropractic in their ignorance and arrogance; they made it *illegal* for chiropractors to treat asthma. Of course we principled chiropractors don't treat any disease or condition other than subluxations, but medicine did this simply to monopolize health care. Ironically, the rationale medicine gave is that they didn't want people avoiding or delaying proper medical care. In truth, this action prevents many people from actually getting well by keeping them away from chiropractors and dependent on asthma medicine for life."

He paused, chuckled and added, "I saw a bumper sticker the other day that read, *Pharmaceutical companies don't create health – they create customers.*"

"And it's not just asthma that's on the rise every year. It's allergies and the entire autism spectrum and ADHD and autoimmune diseases and childhood cancers and leukemia and lots more. They're all increasing each year! That's why I speak out when I hear the nonsense like, *we're getting close to a cure for this or that disease.* Medicine thinks that curing diseases is better than creating health. I don't."

I was puzzled. "How do you do it, Uncle Earl? How do swim against the current every single day of your life?"

"I love every second of it, Adam. The challenge of teaching chiropractic and the joy of adjusting give me purpose and a powerful reason to wake up enthusiastic and grateful every day. Of course, it does hurt sometimes when you run into a parent who blindly does what the medical doctor says and allows his or her child to endure drugs and surgeries that most likely could have easily been avoided. But that's life. As we say in chiropractic, *one spine at a time.* Peoples' belief in medicine often borders on the religious, with powerful emotional ties. To suggest anything outside their medical box of thinking is utter blasphemy."

Aunt Cathy called us in for dinner.

The opposite of courage in our society
is not cowardice, it is conformity.

Rollo May

11

Inside I greeted my two cousins, Megan and Emily, and Megan's husband, Jim. There were big smiles, warm hugs, and lots of love all around. Aunt Cathy served a great meal while Uncle Earl poured some water and wine for us. When we were all seated, Uncle Earl held up his glass of wine and said, "To Adam Hale, may he be the finest doctor the world has ever known."

We toasted, and then Emily asked about my time with Uncle Earl. "Has he been teaching you some chiropractic, Adam?" she asked.

I laughed. "Non-stop," I answered.

Uncle Earl laughed and said, "Hey, if you're going to be a great doctor, you've got to understand chiropractic and the roles of the spine and nervous system in health and disease."

I smiled and said to Emily, "I've wanted to ask him more about his views on vaccines since this morning. Is it true you and Megan never received *any* vaccines?"

Emily had dark-blue eyes, darker than the rest of us Hales. She was tall and fit, with long blond hair and a very strong, athletic-type body. She had a quick wit and was never afraid to speak her mind. "Not a one," she answered very matter-of-factly. "And look, I'm still alive," she added with a cute and slightly mocking tone. "I'm sorry, Adam. I'm sure being the son of a pediatrician, you've had every vaccine that's come along, and I don't mean to judge too harshly. It's just that med-heads – that's what I call people who have an imbalanced and overzealous love, belief and trust in medicine – sometimes think we're crazy as loons for not blindly submitting to the glut of vaccines out there today, so I like to tease a bit."

I knew my family's odd sense of humor, so I nodded in understanding and then said, "Some, like my dad, think that you're only safe because the rest of us have been vaccinated."

Her expression grew serious. "Well, we think we're safe because we have immune systems that have developed and evolved over tens of thousands of years, and that those immune systems are wiser than the limited knowledge of humans. B.J. Palmer, the developer of chiropractic, always taught that our innate intelligence is a lot smarter than our educated intelligence, and I believe that. And you know what else, Adam? I believe it's a lot healthier to go through life confident in the power and wisdom of your God-given body and mind, rather than fearful that the bad germs are going to get you, and that you're in grave danger if you don't inject all these things into your bloodstream your entire life."

I stated boldly, "Some say that the unvaccinated put us all at greater risk of disease."

Emily smiled wryly at me. "Another attempt to manipulate us through fear. Adam, if you believe that the vaccine protects you and your children, then why fear that your next-door neighbor or the child sitting next to yours in a classroom is not vaccinated? You can't have it both ways; either you believe the vaccine protects you or you don't."

I thought of my dad and his disdain for the anti-vaccine movement. "My dad says the anti-vaccine movement is a dangerous fad generated by ignorant extremists."

Emily answered sternly. "Adam, the anti-vaccine movement began the moment English physician Edward Jenner introduced the first smallpox vaccine in 1796. It's nothing new. Although most initial objections were either religious or philosophical, the bottom line is that we are free to think and believe what we choose. We shouldn't believe and accept everything the medical world tells us because historically, they're often very wrong. And the idea that modern vaccines are based on pure science is ridiculous. They are an experiment, nothing more, and there will always be a segment of the population that doubts and questions them."

Megan joined in. Megan was shorter and a little stockier than her sister, with thick, dark and curly hair, and big, brown eyes, which she obviously inherited from my aunt Cathy. "Adam, I don't want you to feel like you're being ganged up on, but may I say something?"

Megan and I were good friends when we were young. She often joined Mike and me in the rowboat fishing or clamming. "Sure, Megan. And I don't feel ganged up on. For much of my life my dad referred to you folks as crazy for your beliefs. But out on the kayak today, I realized that I've never had any real faith or confidence in my body, and always relied on medicine. And for the first time in my life, I realize I'm not too thrilled with the results. I've gotten headaches a lot since I was a kid. I get a lot of colds and sinus congestion, I have bowel problems, and I've got a left knee that bothers me all the time. And I'm only 22 years old. So please, speak freely. I'm actually enjoying all this new information. I'm not sure I agree with everything, but my parents did teach me to have an open mind." I paused a moment and added, "I was encouraged to challenge religion and politics, but medicine? No way. There was little to no gray area there, so it kind of contradicts the open mind thing."

She smiled. "Good. Vaccines are a highly charged emotional issue. We make it very clear in our office that they are not a chiropractic issue, but rather a health issue and a freedom issue. We *never* tell anyone whether or not they or their children should be vaccinated, and we make it clear that it's between them and their medical doctors. I'm sure dad told you that we don't make medical decisions for people."

"As a matter of fact, he did," I answered.

"That said, we do profess our beliefs very proudly. We believe that our bodies have a built-in, innate wisdom that's more powerful than anything man has ever made or invented. And it's not fanatical, but actually rather simple. We believe that nature is wiser than man. Nature made the earth, the sun, moon and stars, and nature is what keeps life going. The great painter Rembrandt said, *choose only one master – nature*. There's not a scientist alive that can make a blade of grass or turn an acorn into a mighty oak, but nature does it with ease. Mankind, with all its magnificent accomplishments, still seems to mess up a lot, and this is certainly evident in modern, western medicine. And although some may believe today's medicine has progressed to a point in its history where it is all-knowing and great and powerful, it isn't. There's more it *doesn't* understand than it does, especially regarding the human immune system. And yet in its arrogance, it often acts as though it knows all."

"What do you mean," I interrupted.

"I mean that it knows very little about the human *being*. Sure, it knows the physical parts, but what gives it life and how it all works? Very little. Voltaire, the French philosopher and champion of freedom wrote, *Doctors are men who prescribe medicines of which they know little, to cure diseases of which they know less, in human beings of whom they know nothing*. And that was more than 200 years ago. I can't imagine what he'd have to say about medicines' love of drugs and vaccines in today's day and age."

Again I interrupted, "But vaccines work."

"Perhaps. People hear and believe what they want to hear and believe. There are two aspects to vaccines, efficacy and safety, and neither have been sufficiently proven to my satisfaction. How could they be? The escalating, mass multiple vaccination programs that exist today have only been around for about 30 years. And each year, since there are always more than 100 vaccines in research and development, the number of vaccines grows. Coincidentally, each year our nation's children get sicker and sicker. No one really knows the long-term dangers of this program because it hasn't been around long enough.

"So are vaccines effective? Perhaps sometimes. Are they safe? Doubtful. Common sense, along with thousands of sad stories, tells me that they're not safe. How can you possibly believe the injection of live and killed microorganisms and their toxins, animal, bacterial and viral DNA, ammonium sulfate, MSG, formaldehyde, glutaraldehyde, phenol, aluminum, mercury and a host of other chemicals into the bloodstreams of small children is safe? Some of these substances are *known* carcinogens."

She paused for a moment, then added, "If these vaccines are as safe as they claim them to be, why not boldly print their ingredients? Tell us plainly and clearly what's in them. But they don't for fear that people may think twice." She shook her head. "Maybe a specific vaccine every now and then is beneficial to the public. *Maybe.* But the quantity of today's vaccines is irresponsible, dangerous and criminal."

Uncle Earl spoke up. "I'm a small town chiropractor in the middle of Colorado, and I've heard this kind of story from parents more than two dozen times in the past 30 years; *little Joey was a healthy 18-month-old, walking and talking, until his second DTaP shot, or MMR, or HiB or PCV vaccine. The next day he had a high fever or a mild seizure and suddenly he stopped talking or became severely autistic. The doctor said it had nothing to do with the shots.* I realize anecdotal evidence is not proof, but when you hear these types of stories enough, you'd have to be an idiot not to see some correlation between vaccines and serious harm. I met the parents of a two-year-old boy who died in his crib 18 hours after an MMR shot.

They too were told emphatically by the doctor that the vaccine had nothing to do with the child's death. Really? Just coincidence, huh?

Megan continued. "No one wants to admit that the product they create, sell, prescribe or recommend hurts people. But the fact is that many vaccines and medicines have killed and continue to kill and injure. Did you know that the drug companies are no longer liable for vaccines when they hurt or kill someone? In the late 1980s, they lobbied and got the government to pick up the tab for their destruction. Can you imagine? They manufacture and sell a product, and when it injures or kills someone, they're not legally responsible. So *they* screw up and *we* pay for it. And doctors don't take the responsibility either, although there are a brave few that admit that what they are doing is wrong, bad or motivated by greed and power.

"If you have a healthy trust in nature, your body, and in life itself, you don't fear diphtheria and tetanus and pertussis and meningitis and all the other nasty things this planet has to offer. B.J. Palmer said, *if the germ theory of disease were correct, there'd be no one living to believe it.* And the idea that we can safely vaccinate our children against every disease is ludicrous."

Usually quiet and reserved, Jim spoke. "Sadly, the medical community has so much faith in the pharmaceutical industry that they rarely question the logic or motives behind what they do. They come out with another medicine or another vaccine, and the doctors simply trust that it's safe and does what it's supposed to do. But they *aren't* always safe, and they *don't* always do what they're supposed to do. As a matter of fact, many are extremely dangerous, causing untold injuries and deaths. So the lawsuits continue and millions of dollars are paid out, but the profits are so big that the lawsuits don't faze them, and they keep making more. If you've read even a little bit about the process by which drugs and vaccines get approved and sold, you'd question and think twice, too. "

I asked Jim, "Are you saying we should give up trying to find cures and vaccines for diseases?"

"No, that will never happen. But we do need to teach people how important chiropractic care is for their health, and to remind them that healthy people need less medicine and less surgery. As far as vaccines go, I don't care if they produce and recommend 200 for every child, just don't make them mandatory. If we are to be a free society, that has to refer to our bodies as well. It is a great violation of our freedom to tell parents that they must inject this bunch of noxious chemicals and biological substances into their babies, or they won't get into school. There must always be a choice, no matter how strongly some experts believe in them.

"I don't care if they – the AMA and their marketing masters, the pharmaceutical empires – tell us that it's for our own good, or in our best interest for everyone to be vaccinated. I should always have the freedom to accept or reject what they recommend. And because they are publicly traded companies, with billions of dollars and shares of stocks on the line, they will continue to do what's best for their shareholders, and that is to make money. When politics, greed and power affect health care, watch out.

"I don't care if they tell us that 10,000 birds are flying over the Atlantic Ocean and each one contains a deadly virus, that they will reach the east coast of the United States in three days, and the only solution is new ZaxaQuiv, a vaccine designed just for that bird virus. You know what? I still want the freedom to decide whether or not I want to receive that vaccine, and I want the right to decide whether or not my children will receive the vaccine, too. I don't want to hear that pharmaceutical lobbyists petitioned lawmakers to make a law that mandates everyone receive the vaccine. And if anyone refuses, they are subject to criminal prosecution and the state may come in and take their children from them. I would expect this in

1939 Germany, but not present-day America. I expect freedom here. And I respectfully reserve the right to always choose whether or not to inject a vaccine into my body or the bodies of my children. My beliefs are no less valid than those who believe in vaccines, no matter how strong their beliefs in a questionable science may be."

"ZaxaQuiv?" I asked.

Jim smiled. "I made that up. Drug manufacturers love to name their products with a lot of z's, q's, x's and v's because it makes them sound more scientific. It's another marketing thing."

"Do you not trust the pharmaceutical industry and the vaccine process?" I asked.

"Correct. I do not trust them. They push a drug onto the market, affirm its safety, and six months later 200 people are dead from that drug. And vaccines? Are they safe? No. Despite what doctors and officials tell us, they're not safe. You think a baby's little body smiles, sits back and says, *now I'm secure, now I'm safe and protected?* Do you really believe that modern medicine and the pharmaceutical industry *always* know what's best for us? That they really know better than the wisdom that created the body? Their history demonstrates time and again that they don't. But if you believe they got it right this time, that they *finally* know what's best for us, that's your choice. I only ask that we retain the freedom to read, study, evaluate and make an informed decision."

I pushed the issue. "But haven't vaccines done a lot of good and saved a lot of lives throughout time?"

"Perhaps. I've read a lot, and I think there's more manipulated statistics and exaggerated propaganda than genuine evidence of benefit. I realize this may sound crazy, but if there were never any vaccines created, we'd probably be going through life pretty much the same. Sure, you might say that this baby can now go through life without polio, diphtheria or pertussis, but there's a chance he'll become autistic, or have allergies, asthma, or ADHD instead. Perhaps his immune system will be so confused and messed up that he has allergies and ear, sinus and upper respiratory infections for much of his life. Or maybe he'll develop leukemia or some other kind of cancer from the vaccine. Perhaps the inoculations have affected the DNA in his sperm, and his children and grandchildren will be even weaker and more prone to disease. Yes, some medical experts have suggested that all these vaccines today may be hurting us for generations to come."

I smiled awkwardly at Jim and said, "This sure is challenging to my medical beliefs. It's like learning that everything you believe in is wrong."

Jim was gentle. "Not wrong, Adam. Just different. For someone to let go of his medical beliefs is similar to a Christian letting go of his belief in Jesus. It's nearly impossible. Deeply rooted faith is hard to move. Some people have so much faith in their doctor that they don't dare question the drug, the vaccine or the procedure. Not even a little question like, *Hey doc, what's in that vaccine you're injecting into my six-month-old baby?* Or *how do you know it's safe?* I think these questions need to be asked, and the answers need to be contemplated.

"I think it's horrible that so many people just line up like cattle when the AMA, drug companies, and the media say, *it's flu season. Get your shots now.* As if it guaranteed immunity from influenza. Flu season, like allergy season, is a marketing tool designed to generate fear and sell more medicine and vaccines. In truth, there are actually four seasons – spring, summer, fall and winter. But it gets people to rush to their doctors and roll up their sleeves without question, without investigation, and without a thought as to what the vaccine is doing inside their bodies. They completely turn over their trust to the pharmaceutical industry, an industry largely motivated by profit. I think that's just foolish."

I spoke up. "So, are you saying that the AMA and drug companies *really* want to keep our children sick?"

"No. I'm saying that they are so entrenched in making a profit and so powerful in the marketing and lobbying aspects of their business that they have lost their vision. They don't even consider research in areas other than their own, even when those other areas might improve the health of our nation. And keep in mind that they fund a lot of their own research, which is absolutely crazy. Talk about the fox guarding the henhouse. As an American, I believe they have the right to research, produce and sell as many vaccines as they like, but when they lobby in Washington and push to make them mandatory, that's where I draw the line. I really don't care if they think it's for our own good. Do I trust them? No. I trust doctors and nurses and EMTs and drugs and surgeries in emergencies, but not with general health. I think they're way off purpose in that area."

Emily joined in the conversation. "The marketing divisions of the drug companies don't care a hoot about what the scientists and researchers are doing. They're not concerned with safety *or* effectiveness. *Just give us the product baby and we'll sell it.* If anybody can sell something, they can. They have dominated the media for 40 years, and when you watch or listen to their drug ads, they sound like a Saturday Night Live spoof. *You may experience anal leakage, brain damage and death. Ask your doctor if new ZaxaQuiv is right for you.* And yet people *still* buy these products by the truckloads, and take them for years." She shook her head in disbelief.

She continued. "If a plane crashes and 250 people are killed, the FAA performs a huge investigation and steps are taken to prevent future similar tragedies. But medicine kills twice that many people *every single day* and we just kind of shrug our shoulders and say, *yeah, that sounds about right.* The public doesn't go nuts. No one demands higher safety standards. It's just kind of accepted as part of life and part of medicine. It's absolutely insane."

Megan quickly added, "But it keeps the lawyers and courts busy."

Uncle Earl chuckled, then turned serious and said, "Vaccinations epitomize the control/fear model of modern medicine. And although vaccines may only be a small part of the pharmaceutical industry's total income, they are extremely essential to keep people in fear and under their control. Vaccines serve as a constant reminder that we are weak, vulnerable and incomplete, and that they – the pharmaceutical companies – and they alone, produce what we all need to survive. Without their precious vaccines, there would only be 36 people left on the entire planet."

I smiled at his exaggeration. He continued. "They actually believe they can control and improve the human immune system, a magnificent part of our bodies that has evolved since life began. They think they know – especially in the past 50 years – how to control it and make it better. And why control it? Fear. If you don't vaccinate your child, he or she may get polio, meningitis, tetanus or diphtheria and die. Fear is the great motivator.

"Well, suppose I don't want to control my immune system? Suppose I want to let it run wild and free like nature intended? Hey, I'm neither uneducated nor stupid. If I read up on a vaccine and decide on these three factors, I might just receive it. One – the disease must be a genuine threat to my children or me. Trying to scare me by saying that two people in northern China died from this disease does not convince me that we must all get vaccinated immediately. Two – they must prove to me that the vaccine is effective in preventing that particular disease. And three – they must prove to me that the vaccine is safe, with no harmful side effects."

Emily interjected, "Adam, you know there's really no such thing as *side* effects, don't you?"

I wasn't sure what she meant, so she continued. "Life works by cause and effect, not cause, effect *and* side effect. A side effect is actually a *direct* effect from the drug or vaccine. The problem with *every* drug and *every* vaccine is that the effects are unpredictable, so the term *side effect* is used to make them sound small and benign. No one knows for certain the effects of any drug, and I guarantee you they're not always benign. If a drug has the potential to do any or all of these things that they list as side effects, what else is it capable of doing inside my body, and more importantly, how is it doing these things? What exactly is that drug doing to my liver, kidneys and other organs and glands? And the answer is, *nobody really knows.*"

Uncle Earl added, "Medicine had experimented with vaccines for hundreds of years, but it wasn't until the 1950s when the pharmaceutical companies discovered that they had a way to control a gullible American public through fear *and* generate lots of money in the process. America's president, FDR, was in a wheelchair due to polio, and the public desperately wanted a cure as the media scared us daily with stories of more paralysis, more iron lungs and more death. Jonas Salk and Albert Sabin offered their vaccines and a new era in mass vaccination ensued. A child of the 1950s received a handful of vaccines, but a child today is injected with 60, 70 or more vaccines by the time he's in kindergarten. Even a little thought on this should raise doubt and concern that all these inoculations can't possibly be beneficial and safe in a 10-pound baby's bloodstream and immune system. Unless of course, you have blind faith in medicine and vaccines."

"Were people really more gullible in the 1950s?" I asked.

"I think they might even be more gullible and fearful today. Back then, many believed Dr. Benjamin Spock had all the right medical answers. He didn't. People were told that it was barbaric to have your baby born anywhere but in a hospital. They were told that breast-feeding was for people of third-world nations, and not for sophisticated, modern Americans. So they turned childbirth into a dangerous medical procedure, and sold us baby formula, telling us that it was equal to or better than mother's milk. Can you imagine? Sadly, even today there are many doctors and parents that believe formula is good for their babies. And although it might fatten them up, nutritionally, baby formula is sugar-coated garbage and nothing at all like mother's milk."

I defended my parents. "I was raised on formula and I'm fine."

Uncle Earl glared at me. "You're *not* fine, Adam. Earlier you said that you've had bowel problems, headaches, allergies and sinus troubles for much of your life, not to mention asthma and ear infections as a child. That's not healthy *or* fine."

He smiled and put his hand on my shoulder. "Adam, I don't want you to feel like this is a personal attack on you or your beliefs. It isn't. As I said before, we chiropractors think differently than most regarding what constitutes health, but our beliefs really aren't weird. They're simple, natural and logical, and on a clinical, day-to-day, real-life basis, the results are profoundly beautiful. Beyond the shadow of a doubt, both children and adults are healthier on every level with chiropractic care, and Southold Springs clearly demonstrates this. People here are healthier, plain and simple. Roughly 85 percent of this community receives regular chiropractic care, and there's no doubt that they are much healthier for it. Emily's 30 years old and she's never needed or taken an antibiotic or any other medicine in her life. And we have hundreds in our practice as well that have never taken medicine. The reason? They're healthy. But if this is too much for you, we can stop and talk about fishing or something else. I don't want you to be uncomfortable at any time, especially while eating."

I swallowed a piece of broccoli and said, "To tell you the truth, Uncle Earl, I am seriously questioning my medical background, and to some degree, my medical future. I'm a bit stunned and shocked by all I've heard in the past 24 hours, but I'm also finding that a lot of it makes sense. I don't know if I've ever felt so confused, but surprisingly, I'm okay with it."

Uncle Earl smiled warmly at me. "Every new parent acknowledges the little miracle in their arms. But if you really marvel at the magnificence of the human body and its creation, why would you choose to inject so many strange and foreign substances into it? *Especially* in a developing newborn or infant. Where's the love? Where's the reverence for that little miracle? Or is it more about fear?"

He continued. "I've met people who have had to join phony religions to obtain a religious exemption to avoid vaccinating their children. Some have found medical doctors who did not vaccinate the child but signed the paperwork as though they had. In a free society, we shouldn't have to jump through hoops to refuse vaccines. Why? Because we don't all believe in them. And just because our beliefs don't align with medicine's, it doesn't mean we're wrong. All the research in the world has not proven that vaccines are completely safe *or* effective."

I asked, "So you think *all* vaccines are bad?"

"No. In theory, the idea of introducing a small amount of something to allow the body to recognize it and produce antibodies against it sounds reasonable. But in practice, it's a big experiment, and I think it's a very dangerous one at that. The initial experimentation may use rats and monkeys, but the *big* part of the experiment is the vaccination of millions of human babies." He adopted the voice of a showman. "Step right up folks. Never before in the history of mankind have we put dozens of inoculations into our babies' bloodstreams. Let's see what happens."

He shook his head, sighed, and spoke calmly. "Perhaps one or two vaccines injected into a child's bloodstream are relatively safe and effective. *Perhaps*. But *dozens* before the age of three? Unlikely. Common sense tells me that they're playing with fire, a fire they barely understand. Remember, they really don't understand the immune system very well. And the worse thing is that they're using our children as guinea pigs in the process. I think mass vaccination has become more destructive than beneficial, and I think it's contributing to the vast and ever-increasing sickness of our society. And who do we trust to tell us when we've reached the point of *too many* vaccines? If this number keeps escalating like it has in the past 30 years, kids will soon be injected with more than 100 vaccines by the time they're in kindergarten! When does it become too many? Two hundred? Three hundred? And the fact that the majority of pediatricians and medical people in general don't question the sheer volume of vaccines these days is utter insanity to me.

"I believe time will prove these points. Regions in our country where people are refusing vaccines will likely demonstrate far greater health. It's interesting though, 5,000 kids can be injured or killed from vaccines, but if *one* unvaccinated kid gets whooping cough or measles, they make a huge stink and say, *see, we told you this would happen.* And then they use that as the example to push their agenda of making sure *everyone* is vaccinated.

"Vaccines have been around for hundreds of years. Trying to conquer diseases has been around for an even longer time. Sure, the technology and weapons of germ destruction have become more powerful, but the thinking is still the same. That's why I boldly say that a lot of medical people have never had an original thought in their lives. For the most part, they're still siding with Louis Pasteur and his germ theory while ignoring the constitution of the host, the *person*. Vaccination is not original thinking. Suppressing and masking symptoms with drugs is not original thinking. By and large, I don't believe them to be wise and prudent thinking either. If someone has a runny nose, you prescribe this. Diarrhea? Menstrual cramp? Heartburn? Headache? It doesn't matter what the symptom is; there's a drug specifically designed to oppose each symptom or set of symptoms. That doesn't sound very creative or original to me, and that's probably why they have to market these drugs like mad. If people were to take a moment to actually think about what they're doing when they blindly take all these drugs, they'd probably say *no, thank you* and look elsewhere."

I asked boldly, "Well, what do *you* offer in the way of original thought?"

"Aside from everything I've been teaching you this weekend? How about the thought that my body has everything it needs to heal and be well. Give a child love, fresh air, fresh water and fresh food and *nothing else*, and that child will likely grow up healthy and strong. Add chiropractic adjustments to the child's life and you've got all the bases covered. Now his nervous system is clear and unrestricted as well, so his body and mind are free to work their natural best. Without adding anything *to* the body, and without removing anything *from* the body, chiropractic adjustments help people live healthier lives as well as help them heal from many conditions and diseases. I credit D.D. and B.J. Palmer with the original thought of chiropractic, and I think they should win a posthumous Nobel Prize for it."

Jim spoke up. "Jonathan Swift wrote, *when a true genius appears in the world, you may know him by this sign; that the dunces are all in confederacy against him.* Emerson said, *Pythagoras was misunderstood, and Socrates, and Jesus, and Luther, and Copernicus and Galileo, and Newton, and every pure and wise spirit that ever took flesh. To be great is to be misunderstood."*

Uncle Earl smiled and continued. "After love, fresh air, water and food, and a free and clear central nervous system, everything else is opinion, belief and theory. Vitamins, minerals, herbs, diets, exercises, medicines, vaccines, procedures and surgeries all fall into the category of someone's opinion. No one in the world knows exactly how much exercise, yoga, protein, vitamin D or anti-inflammatory medicine someone else needs. Can you tell me what the cells of your liver need right now? Of course not. But your body knows. Doctors disagree on which medicine is appropriate or whether or not a tonsillectomy or arthroscopy is necessary. None of it is fact. None of it is proven science, and none of it is absolute. Like the protein-carbohydrate debate, one expert recommends one thing, and another expert recommends the exact opposite.

"Medicine wants us to think that it alone is scientific and valid, and that all the other healing arts out there are unscientific. I see a different division. I see medicine, along with just about everything else, as symptom-treaters and chiropractic alone as a non-judgmental, non-diagnostic and non-therapeutic approach to health care."

I asked, "Non-judgmental? What do you mean by that?"

"Research has shown that prayer can help people heal, but *nondirected* prayer has been found to be the most effective. This means that it works best when it's not directed or intended at a specific target. *Thy will be done*, or *May the blessings be* are examples of nondirected prayer. The intent of a chiropractic adjustment is similar in that it is not directed towards a specific pain, ailment, condition or disease other than vertebral subluxation. We chiropractors don't judge pain and symptoms as bad, and we don't judge any disease as weak or powerful. We know that *individuals* have healed from any

167

and all diseases. From a purely chiropractic perspective, it doesn't matter if someone has cancer or a headache, or is a strict vegan, or does yoga or runs marathons. What matters to us is, *is there a subluxation present in this spine?*

"Today's chiropractic students are taught risk management and reasons to *not* utilize chiropractic care. They are taught to *not* adjust certain people, but rather to refer them to medical doctors if they have severe osteoporosis, spinal cord tumors or something similar. Now of course there are times when you tell a patient they probably need some form of medical care, but I was fortunate to have a teacher that taught us that every person, without exception, deserves chiropractic care. He showed us that practicing from love is far more rewarding than practicing from fear. But sadly, today's chiropractic students are taught, like medical students, CYA care. Cover your ass. Because of this, we wind up with excessive tests and procedures, the overuse of antibiotics and other drugs, and doctors practicing from fear of lawsuits. And it all contributes to very expensive and more complex health care.

"Every person, regardless of the severity of his or her disease or condition, deserves to have a nervous system that's working properly, free from subluxation. I've successfully and safely adjusted people with severely hardened carotid arteries, spinal cord tumors and just about anything else you can think of. Common sense goes a long way, and obviously it's not wise to put a strong force into a diseased or damaged region, so we work *around* those areas. There are only two factors determining the need for chiropractic care – you must be alive and you must have a spine.

Megan interjected. "One of the greatest things about being a chiropractor is that you don't have to try to be the great diagnostician, the nutrition expert, the pain expert, the exercise guru or the psychologist. You don't have to try to figure out what you think is the best course for people to take. Just adjust. Free their brains and spinal cords and let them figure it out themselves and walk their own path. Empower people to make better choices. People free from vertebral subluxation have an uncanny ability to make wiser decisions regarding their health and lives."

"Why is that?" I asked.

"Because they are more alive," she quickly said. "Their brains are better able to communicate with the cells of their bodies, which allow both their bodies and minds to work more effectively. They are more connected to their source of life and power, and therefore are more creative, intuitive and open-minded. They are more at peace and at ease within themselves and with all of life.

She paused and added, "There's such a huge difference between genuine health and the removal of symptoms brought about by drug and surgical interventions, and sadly, it's totally missed by the so-called guardians of health today, the medical professionals.

She continued. "I don't judge, but we've got to acknowledge that a lot of people just don't care about health. They live irresponsibly and abuse their bodies until they are very sick, and then hope that medicine will save them, or at least help them. They choose to eat sugary, processed junk foods to obesity, smoke, drink alcohol, not move, and you know what? In a free society, people should be allowed to eat and drink what they want. You can't force people to be thin and fit. Former New York Mayor Bloomberg tried to make it illegal to sell a large cup of soda. I know the intention is good, but it's a free country. I certainly don't want the government telling me what to eat. But you know what happens to irresponsible, lazy, sick and obese people? They die young. They're *supposed* to. It's the law of cause and effect and the way life has worked since the dawn of time. Life is about responsibility, and irresponsibility often leads to premature death. Whether it was the person who wandered off and got eaten by a saber-toothed tiger, the 19-year-old boy who rides his motorcycle 120 miles per hour, or those who live on fast food and sugar-laden diets. This illusion that we're going to conquer sickness and disease and all live merrily and blissfully till we're 120 years old is a joke. We are ultimately responsible for our own health and the health of our children, and I believe simpler and more natural is the wisest way to go.

"The actions of some people clearly demonstrate the fact that they don't really want to take responsibility for their own health. Our actions are the results of our thoughts and beliefs, and the fact that millions of people take so many daily over-the-counter and prescription medicines tells me that they really don't want to take the time to think about their health. Instead, they prefer to turn over the responsibility for their health to the doctors and drug manufacturers rather than accepting the responsibility themselves. Medicine disempowers people."

I felt defensive so I said, "But a lot of people *have* to take daily medicine to live."

Uncle Earl smiled a bit sadly and asked, "Do they really, Adam? Or is that just what we've been led to believe? Is it really the daily intake of medicines that keeps people alive, or have we just bought into the fear of what *might* happen if we *don't* take the medicine? Now I'm not a medical doctor, so I can't say what medicine someone needs and when they need it, but do you mean to tell me that *every* prescription written every day is beneficial and necessary?"

I shrugged and said, "I guess not."

"Of course it isn't. Prescription medicines injure and kill people every day, not to mention the countless addicts created daily. And these are facts, not unnecessary criticisms of medicine. Are you aware of the times in modern history when doctors went on strike?"

"No", I answered.

"In 1976 in Columbia, doctors went on a 52-day strike and the death rate went down 35 percent. That same year, Los Angeles doctors went on strike to protest rising malpractice premiums, and the death rate dropped 18 percent. In 1973, Israeli doctors went on strike for one month and the death rate reportedly dropped 50 percent. The only time that happened before was 20 years prior, the last time the doctors went on strike.

Uncle Earl continued. "The control/fear model does not work when health is the objective. Chiropractic, at its essence, is diametrically opposed to the control/fear model. Chiropractic is about love, freedom and trust. Love of the body. Love of life and love of health. Freedom from vertebral subluxation and its devastating effects. Freedom of the central nervous system. And trust in the power that made the body. Trust in the wisdom that gave us the greatest gift of all – life. Trust that we are born with everything we need to survive and thrive.

"I think life is better when you consciously accept the responsibility for your own health, and that means choosing whether or not to receive a vaccine or take a medicine. Diseases are risky, but so are medicines, surgeries and vaccines. Being alive is a risk, and no one gets out alive. Everybody dies. And unless you're fortunate enough to live 85 or 90 healthy, vibrant years and then get hit by a bus, almost everyone gets sick at one point or another. Fear of sickness and death permeate society. Modern medicine has fooled us into believing that if you do everything medical authorities say, receive every vaccine and every booster recommended, and take medicines for all your pains, symptoms and conditions, you'll live a long and fruitful life. It's simply not true. But I *do* see that those who consciously move their bodies, eat well, get regular chiropractic care, and *don't* take all these vaccines and daily medicines, live much healthier lives on every level."

I interjected, "But our life expectancy is longer now than ever before."

Emily smiled and put her hand on my shoulder. "Adam, you volunteered in a nursing home, didn't you? How healthy were the people in there?"

I got the point. "Not very," I said.

She continued. "I feel sorry for people who think longevity is the answer. I think quality of life far outweighs longevity, and I would rather have 75 healthy, happy and love-filled years than live to be 90, with the last 15 years sick, feeble and miserable ones. And if the majority of these people in nursing homes and hospitals today are examples of longevity, I'll take death. Many have no minds left, while others have bodies that can't get out of a wheelchair, chew real food or even lift up their own heads. It's very sad, and we don't claim to have all the answers, but we do know that chiropractic care throughout life would have helped the bodies, minds and lives of a great number of these poor folks. Regarding longevity, a wise person once said that it's not the numbers on your tombstone that matter, but the dash in between them."

Uncle Earl chuckled loudly. "And speaking of tombstones and longevity, I wish we had the time to walk through a cemetery this weekend. Adam, I challenge you to walk through any older cemetery in the country, urban or rural. I guarantee you'll see lots of tombstones that read something like, *John Smith – born 1800, died 1892. Mary Smith – born 1802, died 1897.* Sure, little Billy Smith may have died at two of pneumonia or tuberculosis, so the *average* lifespan may have been 35. But don't be fooled – people have lived into their 80s and 90s for centuries. Our second president, John Adams, lived 90 years. Thomas Jefferson lived 83 years, James Madison, 85, and John Quincy Adams, 80. They were all born in the 1700s, and they all lived long lives without vaccines and drugs, if you can imagine that.

"Much of the increase in longevity is due to antibiotics and improvements in basic hygiene. Antibiotics obviously save and prolong many lives, and indoor plumbing and waste removal have also made a huge difference. And although medicine may allow more people to live *with* their conditions and diseases today, I think we're just sold the lie that we're living longer due to modern medicine. It's a marketing tool designed to keep us excited and thinking, *they're doing a fine job.* Again, they need to be in control, so they will influence the media to tell us that due to mass vaccination and modern medicine, we're all living longer and healthier. But the reality is that we're getting sicker every day."

Emily added, "Could you imagine life on Earth if we all lived to be 120 years old? We'd be wall-to-wall people. It would be hell on Earth, and I think most of us would welcome death at that point. Every living creature has a lifespan built into its DNA. Some insects live just a day or two. Dogs and cats live 10 to 20 years. Elephants and some tortoises may live for 70 to 100 years or more, and some trees live for hundreds of years. But every living thing dies. To think we can avoid or prevent death is foolish and arrogant. The attempts at destroying these disease-causing agents only disrupt the balance of nature and make our lives less healthy. Hell, antibiotic-resistant bacteria alone kill 20,000 people every year, another effect of modern medicine."

Defensively I said, "It seems that you enjoy bashing medicine. I don't think that's very productive, especially when you say your objective is to teach chiropractic."

Uncle Earl nodded sympathetically. "My mother taught me at a very young age that you don't build yourself up by putting others down, and I believe that. Medicine has saved the lives of some of our family, and I am forever grateful. I love and respect my family and friends in medicine, and I agree with you that criticizing medicine doesn't boost chiropractic. And yes, my objective *is* to teach chiropractic. I'm not here to bash medicine, but I do think it's important to point out flaws in its rhetoric, logic and science, as well as the fact that it has brainwashed us into a drug-dependent, sick-thinking society. When medical professionals claim health as their objective, yet do things to the contrary, the hypocrisy bothers me and I cannot be silent. This is why I address the pediatricians and their excessive love of vaccines and antibiotics, the obstetricians for their aggressive and sometimes extremely forceful births, and the orthopedists for missing the relationship of the spine and pelvis to all the other joints of the body. I also understand that the men and women in these professions are doing the very best they can with what they know, and that they too help and save lives every day."

"I haven't heard you mention the obstetricians until now. You pick on them, too?"

Uncle Earl frowned at me. "Pick on them? I'm not here to pick on anyone. I'm here to enlighten and educate. Birth trauma is a huge cause of subluxation, and some obstetricians are extremely rough when delivering delicate newborns. I've seen videos of *natural* childbirths that are so violent they would make your skin crawl. One showed a doctor turning a baby's head 180 degrees! The newborn's nose was directly lined up between his shoulder blades while the doctor pulled with tremendous force. Obstetric nurses have told me horror stories of the violence they've witnessed during some deliveries.

"Most people are completely unaware that spinal cord and brain stem injuries are often the direct results of birth trauma. Abraham Towbin, M.D., of Harvard University, has performed thousands of autopsies on stillbirths, SIDS and crib deaths. He's seen dislocated and broken necks, clavicles and jaws. He's documented severed spinal cords, hemorrhage from ruptured blood vessels, decerebration and even decapitation. He found that cerebral palsy, epilepsy, respiratory depression and mental retardation were often direct results of birth trauma. He discovered that 90-120 pounds of force on a newborn's neck is enough to cause instant death, and that some obstetricians *routinely* use that much force when pulling a baby out of the birth canal. So some babies die at birth, some a few days later, and some weeks later, but a big percentage of these tragic deaths is from spinal cord injuries sustained during the birth process. Rarely are the parents told about birth trauma. Instead, they are told that they are the unfortunate victims of a stillbirth, SIDS or crib death. Just unlucky. Obviously, most of us survive the birth experience, but so many of us are subluxated and weakened from it. So yeah, I'm compelled to shed some light on obstetricians and the birth process, too."

Aunt Cathy added, "Birth trauma is a major reason why it's so important for newborns to get their spines checked by a chiropractor as soon as possible."

Uncle Earl spoke seriously. "Adam, did you know that almost half of the millions of visits to pediatricians in this country every year are for kids with ear, sinus and upper respiratory infections? These poor kids are treated with antibiotics and other drugs, and return to the pediatrician time and again. They rarely, if ever, get to experience vibrant health. Instead, they usually get a lifetime of weakness, illness, recurring infections and medications. And you know what current research teaches us? That giving a child an antibiotic almost *guarantees* a secondary infection or a recurrence of the original problem."

He stroked his beard and continued, "Let's say you've got transmission trouble with your pickup truck. You bring it to a specialist and he fixes it, but a few weeks later the transmission goes bad again with the same problem. How many times would you keep bringing it back to the same mechanic? Or another mechanic who does the same things as the first one? Wouldn't you think only a fool would bring his truck back to the same mechanic five, six or more times? And yet people bring their child repeatedly to the same pediatrician over and over. Dozens of repeat visits for the same problem. This is why the medical monopoly of health care is dangerous. People keep bringing their kids back to the pediatricians, and they keep getting the same results – failure and sickness. Chiropractic could likely turn 80 percent of these kids' lives around and give them years of dynamic and genuine health, but most pediatricians and parents don't know this yet."

After dinner and clean-up, we agreed to meet at the fireworks at nine o'clock. Megan, Emily and Jim left for their homes, and Uncle Earl and I retired to the deck chairs.

Paradoxically, freedom comes from obedience to the natural order.

John Heider

12

"Adam, I'd like to teach you more about vertebral subluxation, if I may. And then we'll just talk a little more chiropractic philosophy, okay?"

"Sure, Uncle Earl."

"This may be a bit meaty, but it's important that you understand that one little spinal lesion or derangement, what we call a subluxation, can cause a complex variety of problems."

He took a deep breath, exhaled loudly and began. "Science has demonstrated five major components of subluxation. When there is subluxation present in the spine, these are the results: One – kinesiopathology, which means stuck joints, loose joints, loss of joint play, dynamic misalignments, and compensation reactions. The latter means that when one vertebra is stuck, the ones above and/or below it often become hypermobile in response. This is very common in both the cervical and lumbar spines, and one of the major reasons these areas are often the first to show signs of degeneration.

"Two – neuropathology. Some subluxations are compressive lesions, which is basically a pinched nerve, while others are facilitative lesions, which is a pulling, stretching or twisting of the spinal cord and meningeal system. These don't actually pinch nerves, but rather irritate the brain and spinal cord. The facilitative subluxation appears subtler, yet has been found to be more common and far more devastating to the nervous system, probably because it disrupts the flow of cerebrospinal fluid and diminishes brain function."

He looked at me as though he wondered how far he could go with this information, and continued. "Do you know about the autonomic nervous system and its sub-divisions, sympathetic and parasympathetic?"

I remembered some basic neurology. "The sympathetic is the fight-or-flight response, isn't it?"

He smiled. "Yes. The autonomic nervous system is that part of us that controls all the automatic functions of the body. The fight-or-flight response is a life-saving mechanism built into all mammals. If we suddenly saw a grizzly bear running at us, our nervous systems would change in a fraction of a second to the sympathetic or fight-or-flight response. Blood pressure, blood sugar and adrenaline levels, and dilation of blood vessels all change almost instantly to hopefully save our lives. Now let me ask you a question; in those seconds after we spot the grizzly bear coming towards us, do you think the body cares about digesting the eggs we had for breakfast? Do you think it's interested in sex, hormone production or bowel function?" Before I could answer, he said, "Of course it isn't. Our lives are in danger, and that's all that matters at that moment in time. Organ and gland function all fall under the *parasympathetic* portion of the nervous system, and this is where our nervous systems should be 99.9 percent of the time because our lives are relatively safe these days. Picture a lion after he's eaten half an antelope. He's lazy, relaxed and just wants to lie down to digest his meal."

He took a deep, slow breath and continued. "Subluxations cause disruption and confusion in the nervous system. Subluxated people often get stuck in a sympathetic pattern, which means their nervous systems are acting like they're in danger all the time. These people are often nervous, anxious, depressed, overwhelmed and stressed out. Their organs and glands malfunction due to this excessive sympathetic stimulation, so they commonly have all kinds of internal problems. Remember me telling you of your subluxations? The pelvic imbalance and the atlas subluxation in your upper neck?"

I didn't know where he was going with this, but answered, "Yes."

"People get subluxated anywhere in the spinal column, but subluxations are found most commonly in the upper neck and the sacrum and pelvis – the top and bottom. Now follow this; the parasympathetic nerve supply to organs and glands comes from the top and bottom of the spine – cranio-sacral. So by correcting upper cervical and sacral subluxations, chiropractors actually *stimulate* the parasympathetic division of the autonomic nervous system, which means we *stimulate* the body to relax and to greater levels of ease. Yes, I realize the wording is funny, but the concept is serious. Chiropractic's goal is to normalize the nervous system – to bring it into a neutral and balanced state – *ease*. And hopefully by now, you understand that *everything* in the body and mind works better with ease. Ease is an essential aspect of health, and I've never met anyone who couldn't use more of it in his or her life. So, when I talk about healing with ease, it doesn't necessarily mean *easy*. It means we seek the desired state of ease, which creates an environment more conducive to healing.

"Okay, let's get back to those five components of subluxation. Three – myopathology, which manifests as muscle spasms, muscle weakness and fibrosis. You've heard of fibromyalgia, haven't you?"

"Sure. My aunt's been diagnosed with it."

"Well, break it down. *Fibro* means fibrous infiltration, which is scar tissue. *Myo* means muscle, and *algia* means pain. So, we've got fibrous scar tissue in muscles causing pain. What might cause that?"

"Subluxation?"

"Good guess." We both laughed. He said, "I saw an ad on TV the other day promoting a drug for fibromyalgia. The voice-over said, *fibromyalgia may be the result of over-stimulated nerves.* Hmmm… I wonder what might cause nerves to be stimulated too much. And there's that *may be* again, meaning we don't know the cause of yet another disease.

"Four – histopathology. *Histo* means cell. This manifests as inflammation of joints and soft tissues, changes in blood supply, swelling and edema, and degeneration of joints, cartilage, ligaments, discs and nerves.

"And five – pathology. Spinal degeneration and regeneration, which lead directly to arthritis, rigidity, fixation and fusion. Organs, glands and systems are weakened, as well as attitude, emotions, consciousness, thinking and healing ability.

"Radiologists use different terminology when describing the damage caused by vertebral subluxation. Degenerative disc disease. Degenerative joint disease. Arthritis. Arthrosis. Spondylosis. Narrowing. Central canal stenosis. Lateral foraminal stenosis. Hypertrophy. Osteophyte formation. Spur formation. Uncovertebral arthropathy. Disc bulging. Disc herniation. Nerve root compression, and dozens of others. They're all terms that describe the long-term damaging effects of the subluxation degeneration process. Lots of different names, but all part of the same picture. When your doctor diagnoses you with one or more of these terms, he's really telling you – without knowing it – that you've been subluxated for a long time. And if he's wise, he'll tell you to get your children and grandchildren to a chiropractor so they don't end up in the mess you're in.

"Do you see why we in chiropractic say that subluxation is the precursor to *dis*-ease, which is an obvious precursor to disease? The diminished ease, coordination and control over the body brought about by a simple subluxation can lead directly to the malfunction of organs, glands and systems, which is disease."

I interrupted. "I read that some early chiropractors claimed that subluxation was the ultimate cause of *all* disease. Do you believe that?"

"Most actually claimed that subluxation caused *dis-ease*, not disease. But no, I don't agree with that. There are simply too many factors regarding disease and the human body, especially today with all the changes we've made to our air, water, soil and food qualities. Genetics, environment, consciousness, stress, trauma, diet, lifestyle and experience all play a part in sickness and disease. But our inner constitution is a huge factor, and chiropractic's objective is to keep *that* as strong as possible, regardless of all other factors.

"Being a part of someone's healing from a specific disease is certainly rewarding, but some of the most satisfying times in my office have been when a child's personality changes after an adjustment or two. This is a different kind of healing. I've seen cranky, sullen kids turn into happy ones overnight. I've even had family members come into the office demanding to know how a chiropractor could have such a positive effect on the behavior of their loved one. To see a child go from a raging bull to *I love you, mommy,* is absolutely wonderful. One gentleman asked me, after his seven-year-old grandson had changed into a happy child after one adjustment, *how does cracking a kid's back have anything to do with his personality or happiness?* I took a few minutes to teach him about chiropractic and subluxation, but he left the office still scratching his head in disbelief. And don't forget, it's not me that's so great, and not even chiropractic. It's life. *Life* is what does the healing. Always.

"A few years ago, I adjusted a medical doctor with a huge herniated disc in his thoracic spine. He had severe pain for years that drugs, injections and physical therapy couldn't abate. One chiropractic adjustment and his pain was gone. Completely. Did that disc magically go back into place and heal? No. He had another MRI months later and the disc was still herniated. It actually looked exactly like it did before the adjustment. He didn't care, as long as he didn't have the pain anymore. I recommended more care, but another medical doctor told him that it was a permanent injury, and he believed that doctor, so he never got adjusted again."

I was curious. "So if the disc appeared no better after the adjustment, why was he out of pain?"

"Great question, Adam. I don't know. I guess the dynamics of the subluxated region improved even though it appeared no different on x-ray or MRI. One reason many chiropractors don't see great objective changes in their patients' spines is because they are adjusting adults whose spines, postures and tones have adapted over decades to subluxations and the accompanying negative, compensatory changes associated with them.

"A subluxation is a neurological habit. It is a pattern. It is a postural and tonal neurological, muscular and skeletal pattern that does not change readily when it's been present for years or decades. This is why chiropractic care is best when it's regular and consistent. And yes, sometimes that means a person may need to be adjusted three, four, five or more times a week for many weeks, months or even years. Again, we're outside the medical, quick-fix, instant-gratification model of thinking. We're not talking about taking some medicine and *feeling* better. Taking pills is easy. Just pop them in your mouth and swallow. It doesn't take any effort on your part. That's why I frequently refer to it as irresponsible and lazy. Healing is a process, not an event, and although it's a natural process, it often takes genuine effort. Sometimes that effort is simply committing to regular chiropractic adjustments."

I asked, "If people really need as much care as you say, wouldn't it lead some to think that the chiropractor is just trying to boost his business?"

He smiled at my question. "It might appear that way to some. I know many chiropractors who see the x-rays and MRIs and must know in their hearts that the patient needs years of care to return his spine to healthy status, but instead tell the patient he needs three to six weeks of care. As I see it, there are three reasons for this: One

– insecurity. The chiropractor is afraid that people will think that he's only out to make money. Two – the chiropractor is of a medical, symptom-oriented mindset, and doesn't understand the bigger picture and value of chiropractic. And three – he accepts what the insurance companies offer. All these are terrible practices, yet somewhat understandable. It's not always easy to tell someone the truth; that his spine has been subluxated and degenerating for decades and it's going to take years to correct.

"It is for this reason that I believe that chiropractors need a different fee structure than medicine. In my opinion, weekly fees, monthly fees, annual fees and family fees all work better than accepting what the insurance company offers when the objective is getting and keeping spines free of subluxations for a lifetime. Insurance companies don't understand chiropractic and vertebral subluxation, and are only interested in symptoms. The chiropractors that adjust hundreds or thousands of patients weekly, with lots of infants and children, understand this and work hard to educate people about subluxation and chiropractic. Sadly, many chiropractors have been taught or choose to take the path of the pain and symptom-reliever, leading the public to think that chiropractic is part of the medical, short-term relief model. Although chiropractic does give relief to many people, its real benefits are far greater."

I asked, "But aren't osteoarthritis and disc and joint degeneration progressive and degenerative regardless of what's done?"

"No. Although spinal degeneration has long been considered slow, progressive and irreversible, there is evidence that clearly demonstrates that osteoarthritis can be arrested and reversed by restoring healthy dynamics to the joints. Osteophytes, or bone spurs, can reverse, and joints, cartilage and discs can return to normal or near-normal function. I've seen this on x-rays, and I've experienced it in my own body as well. In spite of much research, there are still skeptics in medicine that consider the arthritic process an advancing and irreversible condition. But a little thought on healing should help us acknowledge that the body can heal discs, ligaments and any other tissues. This shouldn't be the big surprise that it seems to be."

He paused in thought and then continued. "About 20 years ago, I met a woman in the post office who implored me to help her husband. He was 55 years old and had been out of work for eight months with two severely herniated discs in his low back. She said it started when he jumped out of his pickup truck one day. You understand by now that hopping out of pickup can't cause two herniated discs, don't you? I'm sure the discs had been deteriorating for years, and finally reached a point of critical mass. Well, eight months later and he was bedridden and needed a walker to get to the bathroom just a few steps away. He was addicted to painkillers, hadn't paid his mortgage in months, and was close to losing his home to foreclosure. Both a neurosurgeon and an orthopedic surgeon recommended surgery, but he refused because a friend of his had been crippled by spinal surgery. A physical therapist worked on his low back for six weeks and his pain increased. A chiropractor adjusted his low back for four weeks and his pain increased.

"I told her how I practiced chiropractic and that real chiropractic wasn't about back pain. She pleaded, so I went to their home to see the man. His low back was screaming. There was so much inflammation that I could feel the heat generated by his injured discs two inches above his skin, which to me was the body's way of saying *stay away from this area*. I wouldn't touch his low back. But I checked his neck and his atlas, the first cervical vertebra, was way out to the right. I asked if the chiropractor had adjusted his neck, and he said 'no' and that everyone just examined and treated his low back. *Well, what have we got to lose?* I thought. I knew that adjusting his atlas would help his health and life, but I had no idea if it would have any impact on his herniated discs, low back pain and bilateral sciatica. I adjusted his atlas, and the next day his low back pain and leg pain had reduced by 50 percent. I adjusted his atlas again once each day for the next three days, and by the end of the week, he was walking normally and needed no more painkillers. The following week he went back to work and has been working since."

"So Adam, do you think I magically fixed the two herniated discs in his lower back?"

I was amazed at the story, but shrugged a weak, "I guess not."

"So how do these things happen? I don't know. I wouldn't know how to heal a herniated disc if you put one in the palm of my hands. And I don't know if this gentleman's discs *ever* healed, but I do know that a subluxation *anywhere* in the spine can cause weakness and dis-ease *anywhere* in the body. Similarly, I've adjusted sacral subluxations and seen sinus troubles and headaches clear up. If you asked me the scientific explanation for how it happens, I couldn't tell you. Keep in mind that science still doesn't know how an aspirin gets rid of a headache.

"Modern neurology studies so many aspects and processes; sympathetic segmental disturbances, pain mechanisms, mechano-sensitivity, sensory bombardment, meningeal nerve involvement, somato and visceral reflexes, and hundreds more. I've read and studied much of it, but I freely admit that I don't understand it all that well. And as much as I respect the knowledge of neurologists and scientists who understand the complexities of the human brain and nervous system better than anyone, they can't do what I can do. I can remove nerve disturbance and irritation created by vertebral subluxation, and restore proper nerve function. Understanding it and doing something about it are two different things. And I'm not promoting ignorance, but one of the simple joys of being a chiro-practor is that I don't have to know all the workings of the brain and nervous system. I just need to know how and where to adjust to set it free. I trust that the wisdom within that body knows more than I ever will."

I boldly asked, "Isn't that a bit of a cop out, Uncle Earl?"

He smiled, chuckled and answered, "It certainly doesn't satisfy the scientific community, but science didn't get these two guys out of pain and functioning again, did it? The American writer and speaker Dale Carnegie said, *a man convinced against his will is of the same opinion still.* People hold dearly to their beliefs, and sadly, their beliefs are rarely even their own. So many haven't given a lot of thought as to why they believe or think a certain way. Parents, doctors, teachers, preachers and the media have programmed their beliefs into them. That's why I believe experience is the greatest teacher, along with an open heart and mind which allows the consciousness to expand to greater levels of understanding. The closed-minded person has no idea what I'm talking about."

He paused to take a few deep breaths. "Here's some science for you. MRIs have shown that some people with huge, overt disc herniations have little to no pain or disabilities, while others with very slight disc herniations have severe and debilitating pain. No one really knows why. There are plenty of theories. And there is a lot of information about pain and sensory messages bombarding the brain causing muscular, vascular and neurological changes, but pain is so unique and subjective to each of us, it's extremely difficult to measure and understand well."

He added with a wry smile, "You know the definition of the absolute *worst* pain in the world, Adam?"

I thought for a moment. "Kidney stones?"

"*My* pain." And he laughed at his own joke. "But it's true. You can't measure one person's pain versus another's."

He continued. "Pain is a gift. It's an opportunity to learn more about ourselves and our relationship to life. To learn where and how we need to change, grow and expand our thinking or lifestyle. It's a chance to practice creativity, one of the greatest gifts of being human. Pain is also a great motivator. To me, the motivation should be to try to understand *causes* and to make appropriate and wise choices. I believe that most people take the irresponsible and lazy path of – *I don't care where my pain came from. I just want it gone.* And there are plenty of medications and treatments available for these people. But my experience has taught me that many of these folks will repeat the process throughout their lives because they don't understand the difference between healing and curing. They think the drug or treatment cured their pain, but meanwhile, the underlying causes live on and usually manifest again somewhere down the road. When you ignore or mask the body's whispers, you'll likely have to endure its screams later on. This is why I say that people who continually take medicines to mask pain rarely get to experience great levels of health and well-being. As years go by, they generally need more and stronger medicines, have more surgeries, and have less energy, less joy, and a diminished quality of life. Their health continually goes downhill until they die."

"Aren't you judging them, Uncle Earl?"

"Perhaps I am. It's just that the more I see people who rely on medicine for every symptom, condition and problem in their lives, I notice that they groan, whine and complain a lot. I see their lack of energy and their lousy quality of life. And in my opinion, you can't whine and complain and have a heart filled with gratitude at the same time. Like love and fear – the more you have of one, the less you have of the other.

"It is for this reason I strongly suggest that people take more responsibility for their life and health. And the younger someone learns this, the better. When a pain or symptom presents itself for the first time, do something positive, proactive and constructive.

Acknowledge the headache, backache or stomachache and don't just mask it. Change your attitude. Change your diet. Drink more water. Get more fresh air. Get your body moving more. Reduce your stress. And of course get your spine checked and adjusted. Find a hobby that makes you happy. Give back to your community. Serve life in some way, even with a simple smile. Get outside yourself. Sing. Dance. Spread a little love around. But keep masking symptoms with drugs, and it's like sweeping dirt under a rug. Somewhere down the road, you've got to deal with a big ol' pile of dirt. And it's very sad; hospitals and nursing homes are filled with sick and disabled people who've swept dirt under their rugs for their entire lives."

Aunt Cathy reminded us that it was time to leave for the fireworks. She decided to stay home, and suggested we have breakfast together in the morning before I drive back east. Uncle Earl and I headed for the show.

In the car, I asked, "You mention diet and exercise. These are big issues to many chiropractors and other health care practitioners, yet you've barely spoken about them. Why?"

"We can cover them very quickly, because most of diet and exercise is common sense, even though they often become fads, depending on the latest research and discoveries. As far as diet and nutrition are concerned, I recommend fresh foods – fruits, vegetables, grains, herbs, meats. Our food should be as close to nature as possible, which means preferably organic. Raw foods are important because they contain enzymes, life's catalysts. Refined and processed foods are like poison to the body and will gradually weaken and kill us, so I suggest people stay away from canned, boxed and factory-prepared foods.

"Hippocrates said, *Let food be thy medicine, and medicine be thy food.* The father of medicine didn't say, *Let medicine be thy medicine.*

"Aristotle said *moderation in all things,* and I think that's especially true with diet. I'm a big believer in balance and moderation, and I think we need to be more aware of what we ingest *daily.* Two cups of coffee a day is more than 700 cups a year. That's too much for some people. And sadly, a lot of people rely on coffee or other stimulants to get going in the morning, and then need alcohol and other drugs to wind down or fall asleep at the end of the day. That's not healthy, and will eventually wear down even the strongest people. Also, we need to be aware of the make-up, creams, lotions, hair dyes, deodorants and antiperspirants we put *on* our bodies daily. Many people work daily with herbicides, pesticides, paints, lacquers, and other poisons. Accumulated toxins in our bodies can lead to sickness and disease.

"There have been thousands of books written about diet, including food combining, inflammation, gluten, pH, antioxidants, free radicals, body types, and even blood types. And although there's always new nutritional research, they're still all based on somebody's opinion about how and what we should eat. I think the wisest thing you can do is find what works best for you as an individual. No diet works for everyone, and our diets may need to change as we age. Also, know that it's not just *what* we eat that matters, but the attitude with which we eat.

"Researchers studied two groups of rabbits. Both were fed the exact same diet high in saturated fats. One group of rabbits was petted and held; the other was not. The petted group showed less heart disease and arterial damage than the non-petted group. This research, and other similar studies, demonstrates the power of love and affection and their relationship to health. Love heals, and the wise doctor knows this. This is why I put love at the top of the list of universal needs, ahead of fresh air, water and food. And it doesn't matter if it's love for another person, an animal or a plant. Or love expressed through a musical instrument or paintbrush and canvas or some other creative outlet. Love not only helps you live longer, but it makes the days you have here so much richer.

"When we eat unconsciously, or while we're working or driving, the digestive process is stressed and absorption and assimilation are disrupted. Mindfulness is about living consciously, or as your grandfather put it, doing things *slowly and deliberately.* Practicing gratitude for every bite of food you take, as well as eating slowly and deliberately, goes a long way in the process of getting nutrients into the body.

"Also, be cautious when a product or salesperson says something like *perfectly balanced formula.* This means absolutely nothing. Perfectly balanced for whom? We're all unique. When someone offers you *the* perfect formula, or *the* secret to longevity, permanent weight loss, perfect health or spiritual enlightenment, hold onto your wallet.

"As far as exercise goes, I recommend movement. You gotta *move.* A mountain lion doesn't wake up in the morning and do sit-ups and pushups. It stretches slowly and deliberately for a few moments and goes about its day. Now let's take someone who drives an hour to work, sits at a desk all day, drives home, sits down to eat, and then sits in front of the TV for a few hours. This guy really needs to counterbalance that inertia with exercise. Especially when there's stress involved with all that driving and sitting. You can't possibly expect the body to work well when it sits all day. The majority of us simply need to *move* more. Since the inventions of the car, television and computer, we sit more than ever before. And as wonderful as these things are to so many, they contribute to our lack of movement and our declining health.

"I think we need to be aware of our body's posture and tone throughout the day, and move and stretch frequently and accordingly. We need to elongate our necks and extend our spines. Again, it's about living consciously. And I'll repeat, most drugs are designed to make us *less* aware of our bodies, when what we really need to be healthy is to be *more* aware. So become aware of your entire body. *Feel* the tension in your neck and back. I mean, put your hands on your neck and shoulders and *feel* them. Feel the muscles, tendons and ligaments. Get a sense of your own body and where it hurts, where it's inflamed and where it's tight. And when you find tight or tender areas, get your fingers in there and work on the tissues, gently, lovingly and consciously. Instead of taking medicine to hide from the pain or inflammation, increase your awareness of your body with your own two hands.

"Move your body. Do all the joints move with ease? Rotate your ankles. Bend your knees and hips. Stretch your shoulders and arms. Every joint in the body should move in its normal, healthy, full range of motion, and if a particular joint doesn't, you need to work on it. If your neck turns 80 degrees to the left, but only 45 degrees to the right, you need to stretch your neck to the right. But don't try to force it from 45 degrees to 80 degrees overnight. Instead, work gradually. Push it to 47 degrees. Slow and steady wins the race, remember? And keep in mind that most structural imbalances in the body are direct results of subluxation, so of course, get your spine checked and adjusted by a chiropractor.

"Take deep breaths frequently throughout the day. Be more aware of your posture. Posture and breath are two involuntary functions that can be overridden consciously. You can improve your posture by ongoing conscious attention. *Listen* to your body. *Feel* what's going on in it. Read. Learn. There's a ton of information available today. Take responsibility for your own health and life.

"In a few years, we're probably going to have new syndromes named for the video game and texting generations. Studies have shown that many youngsters spend up to eight hours each day sitting with their heads bent forward over a hand-held device. Until they understand and experience chiropractic, their spines and health are likely to be in bad shape. And there's no medicine that's going to help them with their forward head carriages and severely subluxated spines."

I challenged, "Do you believe that chiropractic should replace medicine as our primary health care system?"

He smiled and said, "Great question. It should be a *level* playing field. People should always have the freedom to follow the path that suits them best. Medicine's domination of health care only serves those in medicine, and not the general population. So it depends on your definition of health care. If the objective is truly health, then yes. But if we're in a car accident right now, and we've got lacerations and broken bones, do you think I want the ambulance to take us to a chiropractor's office? Of course not. Or when a baby's born with a congenital heart defect? I'd certainly want a great medical team on the case. Medical professionals do phenomenal repair work, and there will always be a need for them. I take my hat off to every individual involved in first aid, emergency and surgical care. So it's not about replacing medicine; it's about people understanding what we do as chiropractors and including it as part of a healthy lifestyle.

"Life is complex these days. There are more factors contributing to sickness and disease than ever before. Travel throughout the world spreads bacteria, viruses and other pathogens. Our air, water, soil and food qualities are much worse than they were a century ago. Toxins and pollutants abound on Earth, taxing our lungs, livers and kidneys daily. So many people live with levels of stress unheard of decades ago, dramatically increasing the tension in their bodies and lives. These are all the more reasons to keep your nervous system and inner constitution working optimally with chiropractic. Parents need to know that very often their child's sickness is not a complex issue, and that a simple chiropractic adjustment – that may take but a second or two – is all that's needed to change their sick child into a healthy one.

"And speaking of car accidents, consider this – people that receive regular chiropractic care are healthier. Their minds and bodies work better because they are less subluxated. Therefore, with more people under regular chiropractic care, there would be fewer accidents on the road because healthier people are naturally more aware and alert. Their reflexes and thought processes work better. Even when in an accident, they are less likely to incur injuries due to their greater ease, flexibility and joint function. And when they *are* injured, they are more likely to heal faster and more fully.

"Also, healthy people take much less medicine, so that would also contribute to fewer car accidents. People on prescription medicines such as sleeping pills, painkillers, muscle relaxants and anti-anxiety medicines cause accidents every day. Why? Because their brain chemistry is altered or diminished from the drugs. The statistics on these cases are not well documented because we generally test only for alcohol and recreational drugs, but I'm sure a lot of car accidents are due to people legally taking prescription and over-the-counter medicines.

"We don't allow people to drive drunk because alcohol diminishes their clarity, judgment, reflexes and ability to respond appropriately. Well, guess what? A lot of prescription drugs do the very same thing. The labels may warn us not to drive or operate heavy machinery, but a lot of people ignore that and drive anyway. Especially when they've developed a tolerance to taking a certain medicine for a long time.

"If medical doctors understood chiropractic, they would want their patients under regular chiropractic care. Why? Because it would make their patients healthier. Healthier, unsubluxated patients respond better to medicine. And when they need surgery, they are less likely to have serious complications, and are more likely to heal faster and easier." He sighed and added, "We can't get all the chiropractors to get the big message of chiropractic, so we're probably a long way away from medicine understanding what we do.

"There's a world out there trying to sell us products to soothe our pains, heal our diseases and give us vitality and longevity. They're all about substances created from plants or minerals or drug manufacturers that go on or into your body from the outside. Chiropractic is not another product, treatment or therapy to try. It's not another herb, mineral, vitamin or drug. It is a *principle*. Chiropractic is a principle that states that a clear and unrestricted central nervous system is essential for a healthy body and mind.

"Chiropractic is simple and it makes sense. Medicine is complex and doesn't really make a lot of sense, at least regarding day-to-day health. Experience has taught me to be wary of complexities because they are usually far removed from the natural rhythms of life. The continual treatment of symptoms alone leads to weakness, disease and premature death. So many people don't seem to realize that they would likely be much healthier without all these palliative drugs going into their systems on a daily basis. When absolutely necessary, yes, some drugs and surgeries certainly save lives. But the daily need for children and adults to take medicine for weeks, months, years or a lifetime? Ridiculous. This way of thinking leaves no room for healing or growth, no understanding of adaptation and change, and especially, little to no trust in the power within the body. Medicine actually negates the wisdom within us, rather than working with it. Instead, it relies on the pharmaceutical industry to come up with vaccines and cures. The monopoly and complexity of modern medicine has turned health care into a battlefield, and we – the public – are losing the battle.

"I believe that medicine has become too big a part of peoples' lives. Never before in human history has medicine so dominated the thoughts and minds of the majority of a population. Prior to 50 years ago, the doctor played a small role in the lives of a typical family. Nowadays, people have multiple doctors for multiple problems, and they are a huge part of their lives. People take so many prescription drugs that they need to organize them with little plastic cases labeled with the days of the week. Managing sickness and disease with medicines has become a way of life for so many. I prefer to live freely, rather than dependent on daily medicines.

"Health is the natural state of mankind. But health is boring. Health is not dramatic. You're not going to see a TV show about health or healthy people. Healthy people go about their lives with relative ease. They rarely miss school or work. They sleep well, digest and eliminate well, breathe well, move with ease, think clearly, smile more, and have more balanced hormones and emotions. They don't live in fear of the sun, pollen, sneezes, flu or peanuts. Their bodies function the way they were designed to function and they feel great 98 percent of the time. They don't take daily medicines for pain, stiffness, allergies, inflammation, high blood pressure, high cholesterol, blood sugar problems, headaches, acid reflux or sinusitis. They don't spend their days talking about their ailments, what medicines they're taking, what surgeries they've had or need to have, and what doctors they need to visit this week. That's why I continually refer to the basic necessities of life – love, fresh air, fresh water, fresh food, movement, and a clear, unrestricted nervous system. By and large, these alone will allow most people to live a life of wonderful and vibrant health.

"Instead, we've turned out natural state – *health* – into a life-long quest. Why? Because so many of us are weakened from birth. We injure our newborns with traumatic births, and then we assault their immune and nervous systems with dozens of vaccines. We feed them formula, a lifeless and life-diminishing food-like substance, as well as lots of other highly processed and chemical-rich foods. When they develop symptoms, which are usually the body's attempt to *express* and eliminate all these toxic things they've ingested or been injected with, we add more chemicals to their bodies in the form of antibiotics and other drugs. And then we wonder why they're so sick, and why so many people spend years and lots of money in the pursuit of health. All because we've lost sight of the natural simplicity of health and because no one has ever taught us that the health of the human body and mind is directly proportional to the health of the spine and nervous system.

"This is why it bothers me that half of the chiropractors in this country are treating peoples' pain, while neglecting to educate them with chiropractic principles. Instead of offering a chiropractic adjustment, they offer people *treatments*. They put ice or a hot pack on the patient for 10 minutes, then a muscle-stimulating machine for 10 minutes, and maybe traction for 10 minutes, and then they might give an adjustment. The adjustment is a small part of the overall treatment, and from the patient's perspective, has little value. To the patient, the heat and machines *feel* better. These chiropractors have chosen the path of least resistance, and have joined all the other symptom-treaters of the world. I guess they fill a niche for people with back pain, but doesn't it make more sense to keep the spine working properly from birth throughout life? It sure does to me."

"But they're still serving people well, aren't they?" I asked.

"No. When you've got the ability to make profound improvements to a person's spine, health and life, and instead you offer temporary Band-aid pain relief in the form of a *feel-good* treatment, you are short-changing the person. You leave him subluxated and sick, regardless of whether or not his pain goes away. And worse, his children and grandchildren are left at home subluxated. That's not serving people well. Chiropractic used as a therapeutic tool for back pain is like a Steinway grand piano used as a plant stand. Sure, it looks great in your living room, but it's capable of so much more. In the right hands, it can create beautiful music, potentially elevating the listener to great heights. And so it is with chiropractic – it can often lift people to phenomenal levels of health. But when the vision of the chiropractor is small and pain-oriented, chiropractic gets lost in the mire of the many symptom-treating options available today."

I interrupted again. "But I read that chiropractic care is now considered the best choice for lower back pain."

"When chiropractic is genuinely researched, we'll find that it helps people with any and all pains, conditions and diseases, because it makes us stronger *on the inside.* The greatest problem with chiropractic and back pain research is that it reinforces the erroneous notion that chiropractic is about back pain. It isn't. And it never meant to be. In the first half of the 20th century, B.J. Palmer documented cases of chiropractic adjustments helping people with cancer, heart disease, mental illness, and just about every other disease you can imagine. He didn't work tirelessly for decades to treat back pain. Again, that type of thinking causes people to remain subluxated and sick for years until they have pain. Hopefully by now, you can see how faulty and reactive that kind of thinking is."

Uncle Earl stroked his chin in thought. "Which makes more sense, to maintain a child's spine throughout her life, or to wait until she's 30, 40 or older, when there's a lot of damage to her spinal joints, ligaments, discs and nerves? Do you teach a child the importance of brushing her teeth at a young age, or do you wait till she's 18 to start brushing her teeth? If you want the teeth to be healthy and last a lifetime, you start at a young age. Well, the 28 bones of the spine and pelvis are a lot more important *and dynamic* than the 32 teeth. You can live without your teeth. It's really simple, and yet somehow chiropractors have failed to teach people this principle – that chiropractic care of the spine and nervous system from birth on often means the difference between a lifetime of health and strength and a lifetime of weakness and sickness.

"To me, chiropractors with a weak chiropractic philosophical foundation, meaning those who spend their days trying to ease and remove pain, are more therapeutic than chiropractic in nature. They are spinal therapists, and chiropractic is not a therapy. At it's very best, chiropractic is non-diagnostic and non-therapeutic. I know this offends some chiropractors, but that's too bad. They have changed chiropractic into what they *think* it is, rather than what it *truly* is and can be. Some spend more time examining, testing and diagnosing conditions than they do adjusting. To that I say that we've already got doctors doing those things. People don't need more exams, tests and diagnoses – they need health. And they don't need more drugs and surgeries either. To those chiropractors that act as nutritionists, acupuncturists and physical therapists, I say the same thing – we've already got people who do those things. We don't need to do what they do. Instead, we need to teach people and help them with what we do as chiropractors, and that is to locate, analyze and adjust vertebral subluxations. This is what will make the world a better and healthier place.

"Please understand that I'm not saying there's anything wrong with any of these other things. They all help people sometimes. The problem is that there is such a small percentage of the population seeing chiropractors on a regular basis because so many chiropractors don't really *get* chiropractic. Their understanding of subluxation and its relationship to health is weak, so they feel they must *do* more to help the patient get out of pain.

"Keep in mind we are always talking about health and healing, and *not* symptom and relief care. To talk of health without considering chiropractic care is like building a beautiful house and ignoring its electrical system. Circuits are overloading, but instead of correcting the circuit breakers and the cause of the problems, you choose to live with less light, no toaster and no refrigerator. Sure, you're still living, just not as well."

I asked, "One gripe I've heard regarding chiropractic is that once you start, you've got to keep going. Is that true?"

He smiled at me and answered, "Once you start brushing your teeth, you've got to keep brushing them, don't you? Wise people find that with regular chiropractic care, they function better, have more energy, less pain and fewer symptoms, and live healthier and happier lives. Once you experience greater levels of energy and wellness with chiropractic, why would you choose to go back to poorer health? And more importantly, once you understand the destructive nature of vertebral subluxation, why would you choose to go through life subluxated? Or let your kids grow up subluxated?"

I was curious. "So if you were my chiropractor, what would you recommend for someone like me?"

Uncle Earl smiled at me as though he appreciated the question. "Lifetime chiropractic care. I'd recommend you get your pelvis and atlas adjusted frequently and regularly, two to five adjustments per week, for six months to a year. After re-evaluating the degree of progress, I'd say you'd probably do well with once a week or once every two weeks after that."

I was surprised and said, "That sounds excessive. Even dentists only recommend twice a year."

"Dentists don't deal with the central nervous system. Dentists repair teeth that are fixed in bone. The spine and nervous system are extremely dynamic and respond to physical, chemical, emotional and mental stimuli every moment of our lives. The bottom line is – how well do you want your spine and nervous system to work? If you want them to work as well as possible, then you must take care of them.

"For decades, many chiropractors have recommended once a month adjustments for their patients, but my experience has shown me that once a month is simply not enough for most adult spines. It's certainly better than not getting adjusted at all, but due to the severity and persistence of many peoples' subluxations, their spines still tend to degenerate slowly, even with 12 adjustments a year. Since the goal is optimum, excellent function, people need more care than that. Some may call it maintenance care, but they are often maintaining a subluxated spine, and that's really not a good thing. I've found that the exception is the person who's been adjusted from birth or early childhood. He can usually do well with one adjustment a month, depending on the stresses and traumas he endures throughout his life. Why? Because his spine had the advantage of chiropractic care from birth."

Uncle Earl parked the car and we carried our lawn chairs to a large field. Uncle Earl spoke quietly as we walked. "We perceive life through our nervous systems. When our nervous systems are disrupted by subluxation, our perception is altered for the worse. Improve the way your central nervous system works, and you improve your perception of the world. Your world is truly brighter.

"Chiropractic aligns itself with the most powerful force in the universe – nature. Nature *is* science. Nature is what causes a baby to be born healthy after nine months of gestation – without any medical intervention whatsoever. And remember, during those nine months, as one cell divides into trillions, there are literally billions of things that could go wrong. But they don't go wrong, and we usually end up with a healthy child. Nature does this with miraculous ease, often in spite of the mother's poor diet or lifestyle habits. Nature is what heals a cut. Nature is what allows your body to absorb vitamins and minerals from food and turn them into new bone, brain and skin. Chiropractic has always stated that nature needs no help, just no interference. And so chiropractors remove interference to nature. B.J. Palmer wrote, *we release the prisoned impulse, the tiny rivulet of force that emanates from the mind and flows over the nerves to the cells, and stirs them into life.* No other healing art in the world does that.

"You can't improve a sunset, or a tree or the moon's revolutions around the earth. So why do we think we can improve a child's health by injecting dozens of poisonous vaccines into his bloodstream by the time he's five years old? Because we've got an industry with lobbyists and a great marketing strategy to brainwash us into thinking we can improve on nature.

"The reality is – regardless of the presence or absence of pain, symptoms or disease, if there are one or more subluxations present in your spine at this moment, your body and mind are functioning less than 100 percent. Like the dimmer switch on the light bulb, you are shining at 60 watts instead of 100. Since good health means proper function, you are not as healthy as you could be. You are not *all* you can be. You are not whole. You are not firing on all eight cylinders. You are weakened. You are sick. And if you don't correct that subluxation, you will continually weaken further. You will be more prone to injuries and illness. Your nervous system will become less efficient, making every aspect of your life less than it could be. You will likely take more medicines and have more surgeries, and your life will be shorter than it needs to be. All because you never understood chiropractic, or chose not to incorporate it into your life."

It had become fairly dark by the time we set up our chairs in a quiet area. I marveled at the number of stars in the Colorado sky and the sweet smell of the evergreens all around us.

"Uncle Earl, do you consider yourself a scientist?"

"Yes, very much so. If biology is the study of life, then chiropractors are true biologists, because we work with the *life* aspect of the human being. We just happen to call it innate intelligence. Although science is currently unable to measure the quantity and quality of life in an individual, we chiropractors know that every chiropractic adjustment delivered to reduce or correct a subluxation increases the life force in the recipient.

"No one has a patent on truth, and no one has all the answers regarding health and disease. Medicine certainly doesn't. If it did, we'd all be magnificently healthy. But the answers don't all lie in drugs and surgery. And again, I'm not against medicine; there will always be a need for medical doctors and their care. I'm against the organized and targeted brainwashing of an entire nation into a drug-based, symptom-treating culture. I'm also against the arrogance and bullying tactics medicine uses to enforce its beliefs. Health care should never be the big business that it's become, and it shouldn't be politicized, either. Good health is everyone's right.

"Einstein said, *there are two ways to live your life. One is as though nothing is a miracle. The other as though everything is a miracle.* His philosophy illustrates that you can be a scientist and *still* believe in God or some higher organizing force or principle. We chiropractors choose to see all of life as a miracle. Chiropractic doesn't claim to have all the answers, but we do understand a huge missing piece in health care. We don't claim to *cure* or *fix* any disease or condition. Instead, we improve the integrity of the central nervous system, which allows the body to function better and heal itself.

"Chiropractic is an art, a science and a philosophy. The artistry is done with our hands with skilled analysis, palpation and adjustments. The science is simple. Subluxations interfere with the transmission of mental impulses and disrupt the communication between the brain and body causing diminished function. The philosophy too is simple. We are all created from the union of the sperm and the egg. The innate intelligence that miraculously created us from those two half-cells remains with us throughout our lives. Its natural expression is health. The purpose of the chiropractic adjustment is to allow the full expression of that innate intelligence.

He paused a moment in thought, then continued. "Noted mechanical and electrical engineer Nikola Tesla wrote, *Our senses enable us to perceive only a minute portion of the outside world. If you want to find the secrets of the universe, think in terms of energy, frequency and vibration.* Along the same lines, D.D. Palmer wrote, *Chiropractic was founded on the principle of tone.* Tone *is* vibration and frequency. This is why I believe music has a great potential to heal. Research has shown that harsh, discordant music can damage cells, and soothing music can actually help cells heal. I've found great power in singing the word HU, like the man's name Hugh. The vibration and tone of HU can bring peace, balance and healing to both body and mind. But improving the tone of the human body and mind through the chiropractic adjustment is a great secret of the universe, and when that secret is discovered by individuals and families, their lives are profoundly and forever better.

"D.D. Palmer also said that the real purpose of the chiropractic adjustment is *to unite man the spiritual with man the physical.* To allow more spirit into matter, which translates to more life in the body. I know it can't be measured, but it's easy to see that an energetic two-year-old has more life in him or her than an old-timer in a wheelchair. The idea is to be more alive, because ultimately, you are as alive as your spine. Healing must empower, and although it may sound like a cliché, chiropractic truly empowers the recipient. It gives more power, more energy to the body and mind.

"Essentially, it's all energy. Matter is actually energy when viewed closely. It's not really solid, but rather vibrations and frequencies. That said, I believe the energy within light and sound will be the future in medicine, eventually replacing our current love affair with drugs."

"Light and sound?" I asked.

"Yes. Light and sound are the essence of vibration and frequency, and will likely show a greater – and safer – impact on the human body than pharmaceuticals. But the closest thing we've got to that at this time is chiropractic, which teaches us that a healthy neurological tone, or vibration, is necessary for a healthy body and mind. Chiropractic is the great link between energy and matter and between structure and function in the human body and mind.

"Recently, researchers in Europe found that the human nervous system generates no heat, which caused them to infer that nerve energy may be transmitted by sound rather than electrical impulses, as previously believed. As a chiropractor, I find that absolutely fascinating, because it coincides with D.D. Palmer's original idea of tone in the human body."

He paused to take a few deep breaths, patted me on the shoulder a few times, then smiled brightly at me. "There are many things we can do to be healthier. We can learn to relax. We can learn stillness. We can contemplate, meditate or pray. We can cultivate patience, tolerance and forgiveness. We can stop smoking, eat less junk food, exercise, or *move*, more regularly, get more fresh air, drink more water and think better thoughts. Chiropractic is so powerful – due to its positive affect on the central nervous system – that even if we continue our bad habits, our health will often *still* improve.

"Life is better with regular chiropractic care. It doesn't matter whether or not you believe the case histories of the autistic, epileptic girl or the woman with kidney failure. Just because everyone believed the earth was flat didn't make it the truth. The principle of chiropractic, like gravity and electricity, works all the time. If your spine is subluxated, then your nervous system is compromised, and you are weaker and less healthy than you could be. Reduce or remove the subluxation and your body and mind will function better and with greater ease, and your health will improve. And when you function better, you feel better, which makes life much more enjoyable. There are many paths to better health. Chiropractic is simply the most direct path."

Suddenly, there was a loud boom that echoed off the mountains, signaling the start of the fireworks. A chill ran up my spine, and at that moment I saw my future with great clarity and knew I would be a chiropractor.